RENAL DIET COOKBOOK

A Special Informative and Nutritional Guide on Kidney Disorders, Medical Advances, Food Tips That You Can Eat To Preserve Kidney Function, Change Lifestyle And Avoid Dialysis.

Chayla Henck

Table of Contents

Description

Are you having a kidney failure and wondering what to eat? Worry no more.

This guide is a special informative and nutritional guide on kidney disorders, medical advances, food tips that you can eat to preserve kidney function, change lifestyle and avoid dialysis.

The actual treatment of kidney disease depends on multiple factors such as the underlying cause, type of the disease, severity of symptoms, and overall health of a patient. Some diseases can be treated successfully, but others do not have a cure. Before we go on, it's important to clarify this "have no cure" part. Just because there is no drug or other forms of treatment to eliminate the disease entirely, it doesn't mean there is nothing you can do about it. An adequate treatment approach can reduce the intensity of the symptoms, improve your quality of life, prevent the need for dialysis, and make you an overall healthier person.

Generally speaking, the treatment usually revolves around the measures to control symptoms, decrease the risk of complications, and slow down the progression of some specific kidney disease. Patients with kidney disease need to work closely with their doctor, who will recommend an adequate treatment approach for their condition and symptoms experienced.

Kidney disease oftentimes induces various complications that are treated with medications such as those for high blood pressure, anemia, high cholesterol levels, swelling, stronger bones. The most important thing to remember is that proper management of kidney disease also requires diet adjustment. In fact, your doctor will also recommend you should make some tweaks in your diet. That's the whole purpose of this book – to show you how easy it is to adopt a renal diet and make some super delicious foods along the way.

In cases when kidneys are unable to keep up with the clearance of waste and fluid on their own, and a patient develops near-complete kidney failure, end-stage kidney disease occurs. As mentioned above, at this point, it is necessary to undergo dialysis or organ transplant.

In this book, you will learn more about:

- What is the renal diet and its benefits?

- What to eat and what to avoid in the renal diet based on the severity

- Shopping Guide

- Living on a Kidney Healthy Diet

- Handling the Challenges

- Five Tips for Slowing Down Kidney Disease

- Easy recipes to prepare

- Image of recipes ready to eat

... AND MORE!!!

What are you waiting for? Click buy now!!!!!

Introduction

Common causes of chronic kidney failure are diabetes mellitus and high blood pressure, which account for about 35% of all cases. 15% of renal insufficiency patients suffer from inflammatory diseases of the renal corpuscles, the so-called glomerulonephritis. Hereditary diseases such as cystic kidney (8%) and kidney-damaging drugs or chronic renal pelvic inflammatory disease (5% each) are other causes. The various diseases lead to different rates of decline in kidney function.

Blood sugar and blood pressure significantly influence the development and progression of chronic renal failure. Even a slight increase in blood pressure can speed kidney weakness along with diabetes. The systolic pressure in healthy people is in the range of 110-130 mmHg, the diastolic pressure is 70-80 mmHg. A pressure of 140/90 and above is considered elevated blood pressure.

However, the reasons for chronic kidney failure are not always known. There seems to be a genetic predisposition, as people with kidney-related relatives are also more likely to get kidney disease. In addition, we know today that obesity and smoking can increase the risk of chronic kidney failure.

Diabetes

The common cause of chronic kidney failure is diabetes. If the blood sugar level increases for a long time, there is a risk of chronic kidney disease. Increased blood sugar permanently damages the walls of the blood vessels. This hinders the blood flow and thus the nutrient transport to the organs. The late damage of diabetes in the kidneys is called diabetic nephropathy.

By damaging the small blood vessels in the kidneys, their wall becomes more permeable. Small protein particles, called albumins, slip through the vessel walls and are excreted in the urine. The detection of albumin in the urine is the first warning sign that diabetes causes damage to the kidneys. The narrowing of the small blood vessels in the kidneys also means that the kidney tissue is no longer sufficiently supplied with oxygen and nutrients, and the kidney cells die off.

Glomerulonephritis

The renal corpuscles are the "microfilters" of the kidneys and are also called glomeruli, which consist of tiny, coiled-up blood vessels that filter salts, metabolites, pollutants and, most importantly, fluid from the blood. Each kidney has about half to one million glomeruli contaminants in the blood that can cause the cells of the kidneys to become inflamed. Inflammations always affect both kidneys and, more or less, all kidney bodies.

Polycystic kidney disease

This congenital renal malformation usually leads to renal insufficiency from the age of 40 years. Numerous fluid-filled cavities (cysts) restrict the function of kidney tissue. In childhood, these cysts are small, fill up more and more in the course of life with fluid and then displace the normal kidney tissue. This leads to renal insufficiency, which often leads to dialysis in the sixth decade of life.

High blood pressure

High blood pressure can both be the cause and consequence of chronic kidney weakness. On the one hand, high blood pressure damages the kidney bodies (glomeruli), so that they gradually fail. On the other hand, with decreasing renal function increased blood pressure, increasing hormones are formed. In addition, there is too much salt and water in the body, which also raises blood pressure.

Impaired kidney function and high blood pressure condition and reinforce each other. In many cases, hypertensive patients are, therefore, also kidney patients at the same time and vice versa.

Drugs

As an important excretory organ of the body, the kidneys also filter many drugs or their degradation products. However, some of these substances can damage kidney tissue. Medication-related kidney damage is generally rare and can occur only at very high doses (e.g. acetaminophen, see below) or in patients with certain risks. Medications that can occasionally cause such kidney damage include:

- Painkillers, such as paracetamol, ibuprofen, diclofenac

- Antibiotics, such as B. aminoglycosides (amikacin, gentamycin, neomycin or streptomycin)

- Anticancer drugs (chemotherapeutics)

- Iodinated contrast media.

Over-the-counter painkillers can cause kidney damage if taken for long periods. Thus, the active ingredient paracetamol from a total dose of 1,000 grams has a kidney-damaging effect - an amount that is achieved with the twice-daily intake of 500-milligram tablets after three years. Also, in the long-term use of pantoprazole and other blockers of gastric acid (so-called PPIs), kidney damage is increasingly being discussed recently.

Improper use or wrong dosage of even hypertension and diuretic drugs (diuretics) may trigger a more acute renal failure.

Diseases of the blood vessels

Chronic diseases of the blood vessels can impair kidney function. Vascular diseases can lead to reduced blood flow and thus trigger reduced blood flow to the kidneys. If there are deposits of lime and fats (so-called plaques) on the vessel wall, as is the case with arteriosclerosis, the vessels can gradually close completely, so that the underlying kidney tissue is no longer supplied with blood and dies. This can also affect blood vessels that are outside the kidneys. For example, if there is a constriction between the abdominal aorta and the kidney, this is called renal artery stenosis.

Blood vessels can also become inflamed; this is called vasculitis (from the Latin vas for blood vessel). Such vasculitis sometimes occurs only at the kidney, more often the kidney and other organs are affected. They often run very fast, i.e. kidney function can be completely lost within weeks. Fortunately, the doctors have very good medicines to cure vascular inflammation, at least in case of a timely diagnosis.

Chapter 1 What Is The Renal Diet And Its Benefits

What is the Renal Diet?

A renal diet is defined as a diet that is low in protein, sodium, and phosphorus. This diet emphasizes the importance of limiting fluids and consuming high-quality proteins, but some patients may also need to decrease their intake of calcium and potassium. The main goal of the renal diet is to support kidney function and decrease the need for dialysis, but in order for it to work, one needs to adhere to it religiously. A renal diet is not a diet fad that comes and goes, and it's not a program one should follow for a few weeks. Instead, it's a way of life.

Renal Diet and its Benefits

If you have been diagnosed with kidney dysfunction, a proper diet is necessary for controlling the amount of toxic waste in the bloodstream. When toxic waste piles up in the system along with increased fluid, chronic inflammation occurs and we have a much higher chance of developing cardiovascular, bone, metabolic or other health issues.

Since your kidneys can't fully get rid of waste on their own, which comes from food and drinks, probably the only natural way to help our system is through this diet.

A renal diet is especially useful during the first stages of kidney dysfunction and leads to the following benefits:

- Prevents excess fluid and waste build-up

- Prevents the progression of renal dysfunction stages

- Decreases the likelihood of developing other chronic health problems e.g. heart disorders

- Has a mild antioxidant function in the body, which keeps inflammation and inflammatory responses under control.

The above-mentioned benefits are noticeable once the patient follows the diet for at least a month and then continuing it for longer periods, to avoid the stage where dialysis is needed. The strictness of the diet depends on the current stage of renal/kidney disease, if, for example, you are in the 3rd or 4th stage, you should follow a stricter diet and be attentive for the food, which is allowed or prohibited.

These exact foods and nutrients that you should take when following a renal diet, will be given to you in the following sections, so keep on reading.

Explanation of key diet words

The following nutrients play a major role in a renal diet as some have the ability to improve the condition while others can make it worse. Essentially, renal diet is based on low consumption of certain nutrients like potassium and phosphorus simply because it promotes fluid buildup within the system of a kidney patient. Here is a brief explanation of the function of each nutrient and its role in a renal diet:

Potassium.

Potassium is a mineral that naturally occurs in certain foods and plays a role in regulating heart rhythm and muscle movement. It is also needed for keeping fluid and electrolyte balance in normal levels. Our kidneys keep only the right levels of potassium in our system, and when it is excess, they expel it via the urine.

The problem is, once kidneys can't function properly, all this excess potassium can't be expelled out and spikes up, causing symptoms like muscle and bone weakness, abnormal heartbeat, and heart failure in extreme cases.

Thus, a diet low in potassium is recommended to prevent buildup and avoid such negative side effects.

Sodium.

Sodium is a trace mineral that is found in most foods that we eat today and it is the key component of salt, which is actually a sodium compound mixed with chloride. Most food that we consume and especially processed food is highly loaded with salt, however, we may be eating sodium in other forms too e.g. fish. The key role of sodium is to regulate blood pressure, help regulate nerve function, and maintain the balance of acids in the blood. However, when sodium is excessively high and the kidneys can expel it, it can lead to the following symptoms: an elevated feeling of thirst, swelling of hands, feet and the face, elevated blood pressure, and problems with breathing.

This is why it is suggested to keep sodium intake low, to avoid the above.

Phosphorus.

Phosphorus is an essential mineral that is responsible for the development and regeneration of our bones. Phosphorus also plays a key role in the growth of connective tissue e.g. muscles and the regulation of muscle motions. When food we take contains phosphorus, it gets absorbed by the intestines and then gets deposited in our bones.

However, when kidneys are damaged or dysfunctioning, the excess phosphorus can't be expelled through our systems and causes problems such as: extracting calcium out of the bones/making them weaker, and leading to excess calcium in the bloodstream which interferes with blood vessels, heart, eye, and lung function.

Protein.

Protein is a nutritional compound that consists of amino acids, which play a key role in various system functions like cell communication, oxygen supply, and cellular metabolism. They are also a part of a healthy immune system.

Normally, protein is not an issue for our kidneys. When protein is metabolized, waste by-products are also created and are filtered through the kidneys. This waste along with extra renal proteins after will be expelled through urine.

However, when kidneys are unable to filter out excess protein, it gets accumulated in the blood and cause problems.

This doesn't mean that renal disease patients should avoid protein totally as it is still necessary for some metabolic functions, as long as it's taken in moderate amounts and based on the stage of renal disease.

Carbs.

Carbs act as a key source of fuel for our bodies. The consumption of carbs is turned into glucose in our system, which is a primary source of energy.

Carbs are ok to be eaten in moderation by kidney patients and the daily recommended allowance is up to 150 grams/day. However, patients that also suffer from Diabetes (besides renal disease) should control their carb consumption to avoid any sudden spikes in their blood glucose.

Fats.

Being in balanced amounts, fats in our bodies act as an energy source, aid in the release of hormones, and help regulate blood pressure. They also carry some vitamins that are fat-soluble such as A, D, E, and K, which are also very important for our systems. Not all fats are created equal though, some are good for our health and some are bad. Bad fats are saturated and trans fats and are found in processed meat, dairy, and other products. They are also found in margarine and vegetable fat shortenings.

Fats, in general, don't pose a risk for renal disease patients, however, it is suggested to limit the consumption of saturated and trans fats to avoid any cardiovascular problems e.g. elevated blood pressure and clogging of the arteries.

Dietary fiber.

Dietary fiber is a compound that can't be digested on its own by enzymes and acids in our stomach and intestines, but is needed for the system to aid in the digestion of our food and encourage bowel movements. They generally promote bowel regularity and decrease the likelihood of developing constipation inside the colon. Dietary fiber is typically found in fruits, vegetables, seeds and whole grains.

In patients with renal disease, dietary fiber is ok up to 28 grams/day as long as these plant foods don't contain high amounts of phosphorus or potassium.

Vitamins.

According to medical and dietary guidelines, our bodies need close to 13 vitamins to functions. Vitamins play a key role in metabolic functions and the normal functioning of our cardiovascular, digestive, nervous system and immune systems. The adoption of a nutritionally dense and balanced diet is necessary for getting all the vitamins our system needs. However, due to some diet restrictions e.g. sodium, many renal patients are in need of water-soluble vitamins like B-complex (B1, B2, B6, B12, folic acid, biotin) and small amounts of Vitamin C.

Minerals.

Minerals are needed for our system to maintain healthy connective tissue e.g. bones, muscles, and skin and facilitate the normal function of our hearts and central nervous systems.

Our kidneys typically expel any excess amount of minerals through our urine as some can lead to health symptoms e.g. muscle spasms when their levels are abnormally high.

However, as it was mentioned earlier, some minerals like potassium and phosphorus cannot be expelled by our kidneys when in excess and so their intake through diet should be limited.

Other trace minerals are perfectly fine when following a renal diet: iron, copper, zinc and selenium. A lack of these can lead to increased oxidative stress and thus, it is important to take sufficient amounts through diet or supplementation.

Fluids.

Fluids are necessary for the proper hydration of our systems in fact; lack of fluids can lead to dehydration and death in extreme cases.

However, in patients with renal dysfunction, fluids can quickly build up to the point of placing pressure to vital organs like the lungs and heart and becoming dangerous. This is the reason why many physicians advise their kidney patients to limit the consumption of fluids, especially during the last stages of the disorder.

Chapter 2 What To Eat And What To Avoid In The Renal Diet Based On The Severity (Various Stages Of The Disease)

The renal diet focuses on more on what not to eat to improve your kidney health. But it is also essential to know what would actually benefit a kidney patient or someone who has renal dysfunction. There should be clarity regarding how much minerals, nutrients, and fluids one can eat during a renal diet.

We know renal diet endorses to limit your protein intake, but does this mean it is not essential to eat protein on a renal diet? No, you should definitely eat about 7-8 ounces of protein every single day. You should have one meal dedicated to protein which would contain 7-8 ounce. It is essential to combat infections. It also balances muscle mass. This is a healthy way to limit your protein intake on a renal diet. The sources of protein are many, milk, egg, meat, fish, pulses, etc. There are other plant-based proteins too like soy, mushroom, etc.

You should eat fresh vegetables and fruits which would be low in sodium and fat. They should not be frozen, because in most cases, frozen ingredients have preservatives in them. Some of the frozen foods also contain seasonings too. When you are picking your vegetables, make sure to stay far away from the ones that have a large quantity of potassium. When you sit and list your ingredients, you would find more things are on the positive list than the omitted ingredients list. So, enjoy the food, enjoy the process of this diet to live a better life.

Dishes a Dialysis Patient Can Order at Restaurants

A renal patient while going through dialysis has to be very careful about what they eat or drink. But does it mean you cannot enjoy dining out? Certainly not, you can enjoy eating at restaurants, but you need to be careful about what you are ordering. There are many people who take the menu of their favorite restaurants and show it to their dietitian and the dietitian mark which dishes are safe for a dialysis patient to eat.

Usually, the dishes in any restaurants are quite high in sodium and potassium, sometime in phosphate too, while ordering you need to ask them if they can cater to your condition and make you a unique dish that is low on protein, potassium, sodium, and phosphate. Ask them to give you a dish made from fresh ingredients rather than canned ones.

Italian and Asian food are safer options than others as they have a little seasoning and there are no greasy sauces. Even if they come with sauces, ask them not to pour the sauce on your food, instead pour it on the side or in a separate bowl.

If you go to a Chinese restaurant, you can order steamed rice, egg rolls, stir fry vegetables, dim sum, etc. In Thai restaurant, chicken skewers, spring roll, pad Thai noodles, grilled chicken/fish, etc. In Japanese restaurants, you can order sashimi, tempura, etc. In Italian restaurants, you can order pasta without the sauce or sauce on the side. Try to skip soups because they have a lot of flavorings.

Smart Snacking Options for Renal Patients

It is absolutely human to crave for snacks no matter what situation you are in. Even when someone is sick, they still crave for snacks. Renal patients have to stay under a renal diet 24/7 to prevent unwanted renal failure. So, how to give in to your cravings whilst being on a renal diet? This solution is simple, you need to choose a snack that is in sync with your renal diet, and that does not make your situation worse.

There are many healthy snacking options for renal patients. Your snacks have to be adequately counted where they would not cross the limit of sodium, potassium, phosphate and protein intake per day. A good renal snack should be less than 80mg phosphorous, less than 130 mg potassium.

Some patients can enjoy more than other patients, to find out how much nutrients you can consume daily, you need to check with your doctor or dietitian.

Here are a few tasty snacking options:

One cup of Popcorn

rice cereal

pretzels

blueberries (fresh)

2 breadsticks

½ of a muffin

½ of bagel

½ cup sorbet

fruit cocktail

2 Fig cookies

one apple

few grapes (10-15pieces)

vanilla wafers

To name a few

You should not go for snacks 5-6 times a day. Instead build a healthy snacking cycle where you only crave for it when you are actually hungry. Do not give into your snacking craving every single time you have an urge for it.

Chapter 3 Shopping Guide

The renal diet contains fresh fruits, vegetables, whole grain items and lots of other healthy options. You can make your shopping faster and easier by preparing a list of a diet food items. While shopping grocery items for your diet, you have to consider following tips:

Plan your regular meals according to the fresh foods and vegetable of the season.

Whole-grain foods, such as whole-wheat pasta, bread, brown rice, quinoa and barely should be an important part of your meal.

To prepare delicious and filling meal, you can use beans, peas and lentils full of protein and fiber.

Buy fresh lean meats, poultry without skin, seafood and tofu.

Buy low-fat and fat-free dairy food items for regular servings

Low-sodium canned tomatoes, sauce, vegetables, beans, soups and broth can be bought for your meals

Low-calorie beverages, such as low-fat and fat-free milk should be the part of your shopping. Try to get fresh fruit juice, low-sodium, vegetable juices, herbal tea and mineral water.

You can also buy low fat dressings and containments.

Portion Control for Renal Diet

Portion control is an important part of the RENAL diet because it will help you to understand the serving size of food, number of calories the food contains and energy of food. It is also important for the management of your body weight. Portion control means the balance of calories and healthy combination of food items. The food pyramid may help you to understand the healthy balance of each food item. The portion control can be disturbed due to some emotional factors, including depressed mood and monotony in food items. The RENAL diet is designed with combination of your favorite food items; therefore, you will not feel any boredom in the diet.

There are lots of emotional factors that may disturb your mood and meal planning. These will tempt you to overeat, but you have to control your portion size by using smaller dishes. It will help you to having filling feelings earlier, and you can measure the serving size with your palm. The size of protein should not be more than the size of your palm, and the carbohydrates serving can be measured with the fistfuls.

Note: The amount of fat can change your serving size, for instance, if you are taking 1 tablespoon of salad dressing, it is equals to one serving, but the low-fat dressing is equals to half serving. You can increase or decrease the size of your portion, but make sure to have a healthy combination.

Chapter 4 Living On A Kidney Healthy Diet

The kidney diet helps you to reduce the consumption of unhealthy food items because you will be opted to consume whole grains, vegetables and fruits. The consumption of low-fat dairy products should be limited to an extent. You can also enjoy fats, sweets and red meat in smaller quantities. The diet reduces the consumption of saturated fat and fatty foods that can increase your cholesterol level. Following are some recommended food items that you can consume, but try to keep eat 2,000 or less calories in a day.

Include 6 to 8 Servings of Grain in your Diet

The grains, such as bread, rice, pasta and cereal can be included in your regular diet. You can consume one slice whole-bread wheat, I ounce dry cereal and ½ cup cooked cereal, rice or pasta. It will be good to take whole grains because these are rich with nutrients and fiber as compared to refined grains. A bowel of brown rice is healthy to consume as compare to white rice. The whole-wheat pasta is good than regular pasta. Carefully check the label of the products to buy 100 percent whole grain or whole-wheat items. There is no need to consume cream or butter with grains because it will make them unhealthy.

4 to 5 Servings of Vegetables in a Day

The fresh vegetables, including carrots, broccoli, potatoes, greens, tomatoes and other vegetables provide fiber. Vitamins and essential minerals to your body. It is important to include almost 1 ½ cup raw vegetables in your daily meal. The vegetables can be enjoyed with brow rice and whole-wheat noodles as a main dish for the meal. Try to consume fresh vegetables, but if it is necessary to have canned vegetables, you can quit salt to sprinkle on them. If you want to increase the servings of vegetable on regular basis, cut the consumption of other meals.

4 to 5 Servings of Fruits in a Day

Fruits can be a healthy part of your meal because these are packed with lots of minerals, fiber, potassium and other nutrients. The fruits are low in fat; therefore, you can consume a ½ cup of fresh fruits on regular basis. If you want to eat avocados and coconuts, don't forget to consult your doctor about it because these are not good to include in your diet.

- You can eat fruits as a snack, or take them with meal. The fruits can also be the part of your dessert and low-fat yogurt.

- It will be good to consume with edible peels, such as apples, pears and other fruits. You can enjoy the apples, pears and other fruits with the peels to get healthy nutrients and fiber.

- The citrus fruits and juice, including grapefruit, organs and lemons can react with certain medicines; therefore, it is necessary to check your doctor or pharmacist before including these fruits in your diet.

- Always try to eat fresh fruits because the canned fruits and juices may contain sugar, and it is not good for your health.

2 to 3 Servings of Dairy in a Day

The milk, cheese, yogurt and cream are dairy products, but you have to be very careful while including them in your regular diet. Always choose low-fat dairy products because these are the main source of vitamin D, protein and calcium. Fat-free dairy products should be included in your diet, such as skimmed milk and yogurt. One serving may contain a cup of skimmed milk, a cup of yogurt and 1 ½ oz. cheese.

The fat-free yogurt will be a sweet treat for you because you can add fruits to increase its nutritional value and taste. If it is difficult for you to consume dairy products, you can try products that are free from lactose. Be careful while taking fat-free cheese because it may contain high amount of sodium.

6 or Less Servings of Lean Meat, Fish and Poultry

You can supply lots of protein, vitamins B, iron and zinc available in the meat, but you have to be very careful while including meat in your diet. The meat is rich with fat and cholesterol, but you can make the meat healthy by mixing them with vegetables. For instance, 1 oz. seafood, 1 egg and skinless poultry. By trimming skin and fat from meat, you can make it healthier. It will be good to eat bake, grilled, boil or roasted meat instead of frying it. Keep your heart healthy with tuna, salmon and herring because the fish is high in cholesterol and omega-3 fatty acid.

4 to 5 Servings of Nuts, Seeds and legumes in a Week

If you want to get magnesium, protein and potassium, it will be good to consume almonds, sunflower seeds, beans, lentils, peas and other food items of the similar family. The food is full of fiber and phytochemicals to protect you from cardiovascular disease and cancers. The serving size should be small for each week because these types of food may contain high calories. One serving should comprise of 1/3 cups of nuts, 2 tablespoons of seeds and ½ cup cooked beans.

- The nuts contain healthy types of fat and Omeag-3 fatty acids and are high in calories. Try to eat moderate number of nuts, seeds and legumes by adding them in cereals and salads.

- Soybean based products can be consumed instead of meat because these contain all essential amino acids important for your body.

2 to 3 Servings of Fats and Oils

Fats are important for the immunity system of your body, and these will help your body to absorb all essential vitamins. It is important to be very careful while consuming fats and oils because excessive fats can increase the risk of various diseases, such as diabetes, obesity and heart diseases. The RENAL diet will help you to limit the amount of fat in your meal. You have to include healthy and monounsaturated fats, such as 1 teaspoon soft margarine, 1 tablespoon mayonnaise and 2 tablespoons salad dressing.

The saturated fats will increase the cholesterol level in your blood and increase the risk of coronary artery diseases. With the help of RENAL, you will be able to limit the use of butter, cream, cheese, meat, cream and eggs in your meal.

There is no need to take Trans-fat available in the crackers, fried and baked items. It will be good to read the labels of food before buying salad dressing and margarine. It can help you to choose lowest saturated fat.

5 or Fewer Servings of Sweets in Diet

If you are a sweets lover, there is no need to avoid it because 1 tablespoon sugar, jam or jelly is allowed in RENAL diet on a weekly basis.

- It is important to choose fat-free sweets in your meal, such as sorbets, fruit ices, hard candy, low-fat and sugar free cookies and graham crackers.

- Artificial sweeteners, such as sucralose, NutraSweet and Splenda may help you to satisfy your sugar craving without increasing your calories and blood sugar. You can use diet cola instead of regular one, but don't forget to check the nutrition of each beverage before selecting it.

- There is no need to add sugar in the drink because it will increase its caloric content.

Alcohol and Caffeine

The alcohol has lots of side effects, including high blood pressure, and the RENAL diet recommends you to avoid or limit alcohol to few drinks a week. The RENAL diet is silent about caffeine because the caffeine can increase your blood pressure on temporary basis. If you have high blood pressure, and it is affected by caffeine as well, it will be good to consult your doctor before taking any decision.

Chapter 5 Handling The Challenges

Handling the cravings

We like to treat ourselves now and then, but don't forget that high-sugar food items, such as chips, cookies, and cakes, offer empty calories with little or no nutritional value. Delicious recipes in this book will satisfy your sweet tooth. Make sure to keep hard candies, gelatin, ice pops, sherbet, and vanilla wafers in your pantry to help you stay on track. Occasionally, allow yourself to have a scoop of ice cream or a slice of vanilla cake.

Low-Sodium Seasoning Choices

Controlling sodium intake is important for people with chronic kidney disease, but a low sodium renal diet doesn't mean your meals have to be bland. Your meals can be quite enjoyable with a little creativity and experimentation with herbs and spices. Popular herbs and spices you can use when cooking pork, beef, chicken, fish, and vegetables include bay leaf, allspice, black pepper, caraway, cardamom, curry, dill, fresh garlic, fresh onion, ginger, lemon juice, rosemary, marjoram, thyme, sage, and tarragon. There are also salt-free blends you can purchase, including Bragg Organic, Sprinkle 24 Herbs and Spices Seasoning, Chef Paul Prudhomme's Magic Salt-Free Seasonings, Mrs. Dash seasoning blends, and Lawry's Salt-Free 17 Seasoning. Always check the ingredient list of any seasoning mix to avoid blends with salt and potassium. Creating your own seasoning mix is a great option.

Dining Out

Dining out can still be an enjoyable experience even on a renal diet. It is all about making smart meal choices and picking foods that are low in potassium, phosphorus, and sodium. Make sure to have a good plan in place when dining out. When in doubt, go online, and view the menu if available before you visit a restaurant. Prepare any questions you may have for the server. Be mindful of portion sizes. An easy way to limit your phosphorus, sodium, and potassium intake is to share your meal.

Or you can eat half of your meal at the restaurant and take the other half home.

Types of food	Avoid or limit	Better choices
Buffet	Soups, chips, potato items, raw spinach, olives, three-bean salads, dried fruit, fresh fruit salad	Salad bar (limit serving size to that of a bread and butter plate or a small bowl), Chinese noodles, grated cheese in moderation, canned fruit cocktail, macaroni salad, fresh grapes, fresh or canned pineapple, small fresh peach, grilled, pan-fried, or marinated meats
Asian	Nuts: green leafy vegetables, such as bok choy, Chinese spinach, Chines cabbage, fried rice, soy sauce, teriyaki sauce	Steamed veggies, rice, plain noodles; request your food to be prepared without any fish sauce, soy sauce, or MSG
Fast Food	French fries, fried fish, fried chicken, ketchup, mustard, milkshakes, and dark sodas	Unsalted onion rings, salads, ask the condiments to be left on the side Taco bell: a taco with few or no tomatoes McDonald's: plain hamburger Burger King: plain hamburger

Mexican	Beans, guacamole, cheese, tomatoes	Plain rice, tacos, burritos, fajitas, and enchiladas filled with minced meat, beef or chicken
Italian	Red sauces, white sauces	Wine sauces like with chicken Plain or meat-filled pasta Order sauce on the side A small portion of clam and mussel sauces 1 tbsp. Parmesan Salad, bread, very plain pasta
Mediterranean	Spinach-filled phyllo pastries, sausage rolls, Chiko rolls, tabbouleh, falafel, scalloped potatoes	Cream or white-wine sauces, grilled, pan-fried, or marinated meats, chicken, fish, or seafood; dishes served with rice, couscous, kebabs and skewered lean meats; risotto
Barbecue	Barbecue sauce, steak sauce, mustard, ketchup, horseradish, sausage, hot dogs, cornbread	Lean meat, chicken, fish or seafood; French bread or garlic bread, grilled vegetable marinades with wine, lemon juice, oil, vinegar, garlic, honey, herbs, and spices

Entrees	Casseroles, sauces, gravies, heavily fried items, breaded or battered foods, cured or salted meats, omelets with cheese, ham, sausage, or bacon	Broiled grilled lean meats and fish, omelets with vegetables, sandwiches with meat filling
Sides	Kale, spinach, potato products, tomatoes, mushrooms, winter squash	Peas, sweet peas, green beans, corn, cabbage, zucchini, eggplant, cauliflower, lentils, plain rice, jasmine rice, pasta, noodles
Desserts	Chocolate, nuts, coconut, cheesecake, custard, puddings, dried fruit, star fruit, cantaloupe, oranges, pies such as cream, minced, pumpkin, rhubarb, and ice cream	Low-potassium fresh fruit or canned fruit, sugar cookies, angel food cake, gelatin

Strategies to Dining Out

Eating at Social Gatherings

Birthdays, weddings, graduations, picnics, and barbecues are wonderful occasions for getting together with family and friends. For people with kidney disease, those social gatherings can also mean tough choices about what to eat and drink. Here are some kidney-healthy diet tips for social gatherings:

1.   Don't go hungry: Have a snack before you leave the house. Going to any event hungry will only set you up for disaster, and you are likely to overeat. Having a high-protein snack beforehand will make you feel a little full and help you make healthier choices.

2.   Avoid high-sodium foods: Salty foods will only make you thirsty, which will make you want to drink more than you probably should. Choose low-sodium foods such as chicken and hamburgers, instead of hot dogs or sausages. You can choose grilled vegetables.

3.   Limit alcohol: It is best to speak with your physician first about drinking alcohol. Alcoholic beverages also count toward your fluid intake.

4.   Food safety is important: Having kidney disease does put you at a higher risk for foodborne illnesses. Keep food at safe temperatures, wash produce well, and use separate cutting boards for raw and cooked meats.

5.   Plan ahead: Feel free to ask your family or friends about the menu. This way you can decide exactly what you want to eat.

Chapter 6 Five Tips For Slowing Down Kidney Disease

Having your kidneys function better for a longer period is one more day you don't have to worry about kidney failure. The more you slow down your CKD's progress, the fewer chances you have of finally looking for drastic kidney treatments. Some of the changes that you use for your kidneys also work to improve other organs in your body, such as your heart.

Just what are the tips that you need to follow to slow down kidney disease?

Tip #1: Maintain Your Blood Sugar in the Target Range

When you are checking blood sugar levels, you might find out that your blood sugar levels go through quite a few changes. It is not important to focus on these changes heavily when gauging the blood sugar levels, but they are important to know if you would like to get more details of your sugar levels. Before venturing further into understanding your glucose levels, I would like to first draw your attention to a particular measurement – mmol/L.

'Mmol' is short for millimole. A mole essentially calculates just how many atoms of a particular mineral or compound is present in a chemical process or reaction. A millimole is one-thousandth of a mole. The measurement is used to make precise calculations of the contents of fluids in our body, especially when it comes to blood sugar levels. The 'L' in mmol/L represent liters. What the measurement is trying to show you is the number of atoms of glucose or sugar (represented in mmol) is present in every liter of your blood. A typical adult will have anywhere between 4.7 to 5.5 liters of blood in their body. By using mmol/L, you get to know if you have high or low sugar content.

Now we return to the idea that measuring blood sugar levels is a little more complex than you originally thought.

Here is a table to help you understand the difference. It shows you the recommended glucose levels during various scenarios in your daily life (The Global Diabetes Community, 2019).

Target Levels by Type	Immediately After Waking	Before Having Meals	Around 90 Minutes After Having Meals
No diabetes		4 to 5.9 mmol/L	under 7.8 mmol/L
Type 2 diabetes		4 to 7 mmol/L	under 8.5 mmol/L
Type 1 diabetes	5 to 7 mmol/L	4 to 7 mmol/L	5 to 9 mmol/L
Children with type 1 diabetes	4 to 7 mmol/L	4 to 7 mmol/L	5 to 9 mmol/L

The above table might seem intimidating. You might be wondering what all those numbers are and if you might require a mathematical formula to even figure out what half the numbers in the table represent. Thankfully, that won't be necessary. The table is actually really simple to understand once you realize the fact that the numbers represent a range.

Let's take the first row, which represents the blood sugar levels of people who do not have diabetes. For such people, the normal blood sugar levels fall in the range of 4.0 to 5.9 mmol/L before they have any meal. Once they have their meal and the food is undergoing a proper digestive process (which helps the body absorb the glucose in the food), the blood sugar levels should be below 7.8 mmol/L. This does not mean that if the sugar levels rise above the recommended levels, then it is fatal to you. It simply means that the risk of getting diabetes or experiencing various side effects increases. In the second row, the numbers represent the recommended blood sugar range for people suffering from Type 2 diabetes. Anything above the range could trigger some of the side effects of diabetes or worsen the condition.

But the table tells you something important as well. Usually, you should make sure that when you are not eating, your blood sugar levels should not increase above 7 mmol/L and after eating, you should keep it below 9 mmol/L.

Apart from focusing on the recipes in this book, make sure that you keep an active lifestyle. I am not asking you to hit the gym and aim for a six-pack. Rather, enjoy the outdoors and go for walks. Ensure that you are not sitting in one spot for more than an hour straight. Perform stretching exercises if you find yourself working in a seated position for too long.

Tip #2: Maintain Your Blood Pressure in the Target Range

You must have guessed that this tip was coming. Well, here it is and it goes side-by-side with the previous tip. Once again, before we dive headfirst into the tip itself, it is time to understand the measurement used to indicate blood pressure levels - mmHg.

When measuring the pressure levels in your blood, one cannot simply say that you have a certain level of pressure. That is because pressure is a difficult concept to explain. It is similar to asking a person to measure the levels of pain he or she feels from various injuries. In order to make it easier to understand blood pressure, it gets compared to a column of mercury. The 'mm' in mmHg stands for millimeters and Hg is the chemical symbol for mercury. Each unit of the measurement explains how much pressure a column of mercury 1 millimeter high exerts. For example, if the reading shows 2 mmHg, then the pressure exerted by your blood is similar to the pressure exerted by a column of mercury 2 millimeter high. Now you can, more or less, imagine how pressure works in the blood. You have a reference point – which is mercury in this case – to work with.

An ideal blood pressure level is when the readings are below 120/80 mmHg. If the blood pressure falls between 120/80mmHg to 139/89mmHg, then the pressure falls in the normal to high range. Blood pressure over the 140/90mmHg mark is considered as high.

Here is the truth; even if you have had low blood pressure all your life, you might find it difficult to manage your blood pressure after having CKD. The diet will definitely go a long way in blood pressure management, but you should still get in touch with your doctor to see if you might need medicines to further keep the pressure in check. Try to check your pressure every day so that you are on top of things and are ready to take action at the first sign of an above-normal result.

Tip #3: Maintain Your Weight

According to the National Kidney Foundation, being overweight has both an indirect and a direct effect on the kidneys.

Here is the indirect effect. Additional weight worsens the cases of diabetes and blood pressure in the body. As we had noticed with high diabetes and high blood pressure, the situation becomes a vicious circle that eventually leads to kidney failure.

Now for the direct effect. When the body has extra weight, all of that weight gets pushed downwards. It makes the kidneys work much harder and filter wastes that are more than the regular level. All of the extra work only adds more burden on the kidneys and eventually, you begin to see the results. Remember this, your kidney has more work to deal with.

At this point, it is important to mention this; being overweight is nothing to be ashamed about. Rather, it gives you a starting point for your goals and helps you decide where you would like to go next. It tells you just how much physical activity you must incorporate into your life in order to start noticing visible changes. Sure, the road to a healthy body is filled with numerous obstacles, some of which are challenging to overcome. But the rewards are worth it. You are not looking to get the "ideal body," "perfect body" or the "six-pack abs." You are trying to get your body to a state where it results in positive effects on your health.

Tip #4: Quit Smoking and Sodas

Sodas are packed with more sugar than your kidneys can handle. In fact, you might just be pushing your kidneys to overwork in order to properly filter through all that sugar. This is why it comes as no surprise that when you have CKD, you should aim to manage the sugar content you consume, not just from sodas, but from other sweet and sugar-filled substances.

If you had been smoking, now would be a good time to get rid of the habit. Don't think of reducing the number of times you smoke. You should be thinking about trying to quit the habit entirely.

Tip #5: Apart from Sodium, Potassium, and Phosphorus, You Should Reduce Protein Intake

When protein is consumed by the body, it breaks down into components called blood urea nitrogen, or BUN for short. The name of the components might sound a bit tacky, but their effect on your kidneys are rather serious. BUN is a difficult component for your kidneys to remove. The organs are not able to filter them properly. The less protein you eat, the less BUN is made in your body.

This does not mean that you have to reduce consuming proteins completely. It just means that you have to manage your protein intake.

While it is important to talk about limiting sodium, potassium, and phosphorus in your diet, the bigger question is just how you can actually go about limiting these minerals. That is something we are going to discuss in the next chapter.

Chapter 7 Recipes

Breakfast
Congee with century eggs

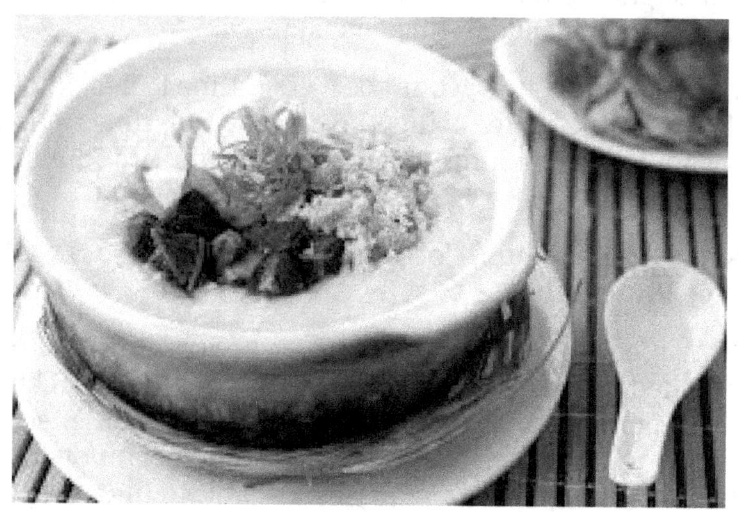

Servings: 6

Preparation Time: 6 hours 15 minutes

Ingredients:

6 cups water

½ cup red quinoa

2 garlic cloves, grated

2 large leeks, minced

1 tablespoon coconut oil

1 tablespoon brown rice, rinsed, drained

½ tablespoon dark soy sauce

¼ tablespoon low-sodium soy sauce

¼ tablespoon low-sodium teriyaki sauce

½ teaspoon ginger, grated

⅛ teaspoon white pepper

¼ pound ground lean beef

Pinch of sea salt

2 large century eggs, boiled, quartered

Dash of red pepper flakes

Dash of garlic flakes

Directions:

Pour oil into non-stick skillet set over medium heat. Sauté leeks
and garlic until limp and aromatic
add in beef. Stir-fry until meat browns
pour into slow cooker set at medium heat.

Except for garnishes, pour in remaining ingredients
stir. Put lid on. Cook for 6 hours. Turn off heat. Taste
adjust seasoning if needed.

Ladle congee into individual bowls. Garnish with leeks and
century eggs. Sprinkle in garlic flakes and red pepper flakes.
Cool slightly before serving.

Nutrition:
protein 10.35g
potassium (k) 267 mg (6 %) and sodium, Na 148 mg

Breakfast cheesecake

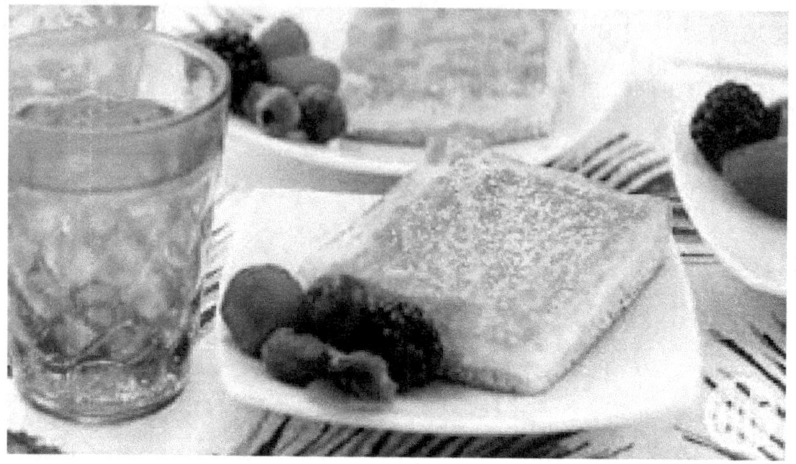

Servings: 16

Preparation Time: 20 minutes plus 1-hour chill time

Ingredients:

4 eggs

7 cups Greek yogurt

7 cups cottage cheese

2 tablespoons honey, add more if needed

2 teaspoons vanilla

½ teaspoon olive oil

½ onion, chopped

½ cup uncured sausage

Pinch of salt

Pinch of pepper

Directions:

In a blender, combine eggs, cream cheese, cottage cheese, honey, and vanilla. Process until all ingredients are well combined.

Meanwhile, heat the olive oil in a pan. Sauté onion and uncured sausage. Season with salt and pepper. Cook for 4 minutes. Transfer the mixture into a baking dish.

Place inside the oven and bake for 10 minutes. Allow to cool at room temperature. Refrigerate for 1 hour before serving

Nutrition:
protein 22.92g
potassium (k) 244 mg
sodium, Na 477 mg

Mock cream cheese pancake

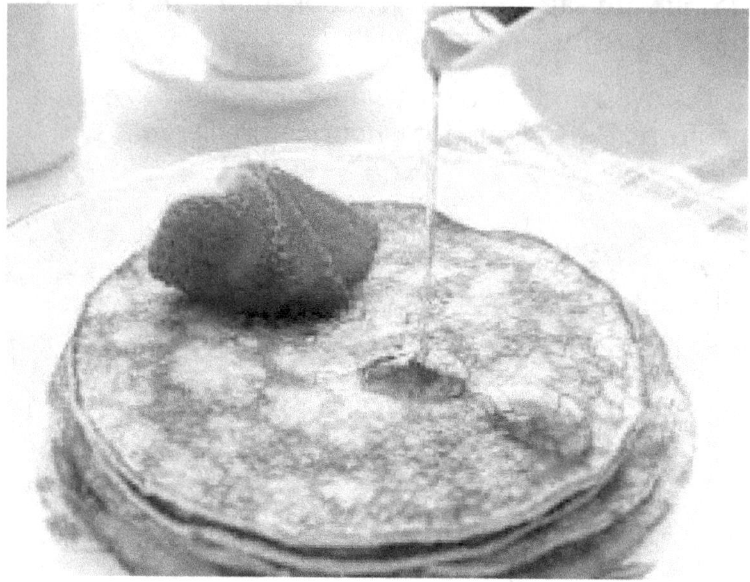

Servings: 4

Preparation Time: 10 minutes

Ingredients:

2 cups Greek yogurt

½ teaspoon cinnamon

2 eggs

1 pack stevia

Directions:

Put eggs, cream cheese, stevia, and cinnamon in a blender. Process until all ingredients are well-combined.

Pour an equal amount of the blended mixture in a greased pan. Cook for 4 minutes on both sides. Repeat with the rest of the batter. Serve.

Nutrition:
protein 13.16g
potassium (k) 199 mg
sodium, Na 82mg

Eggs creamy melt

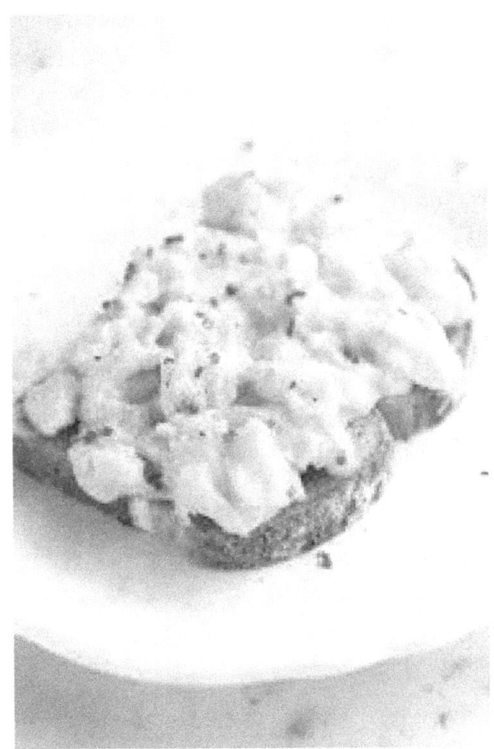

Servings: 2

Preparation Time: 10 minutes

Ingredients:

2 eggs, beaten

Italian seasoning

1 cup tofu, shredded

1 tablespoon olive oil

Directions:

In a small bowl, combine beaten eggs and Italian seasoning
Sprinkle tofu on top.

Heat the olive oil in a pan. Add the egg mixture. Cook for 4 minutes on both sides. Serve.

Nutrition:
protein 15.57g
potassium (k) 216 mg
sodium, Na 107 mg

Mashed cauliflowers

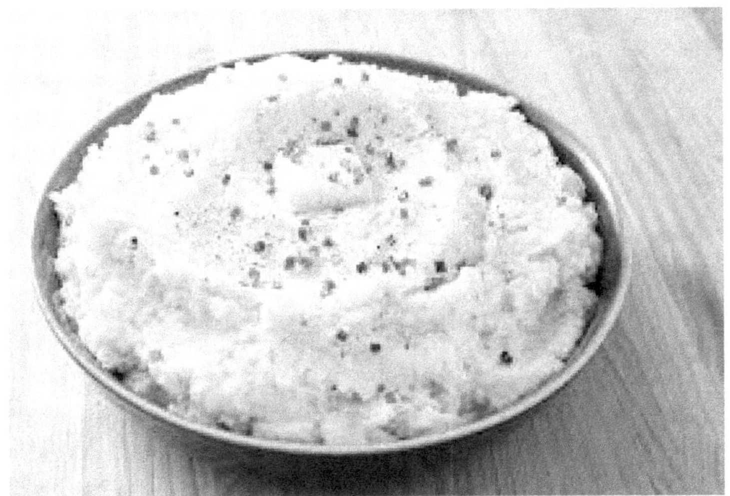

Servings: 1

Preparation Time: 10 minutes

Ingredients:

1 cup cauliflower florets

2 tablespoons unsalted butter

¼ cup sour cream

Pinch of pepper

Directions:

Steam cauliflower florets for 5 minutes or until soft.

Process steamed florets in a food processor.

Add in butter and sour cream. Process again until all ingredients are well combined. Serve.

Nutrition:
protein 4.24g
potassium (k) 448 mg
sodium, Na 204 mg
 - with unsalted butter content of sodium is 83 mg

Pistachios salad

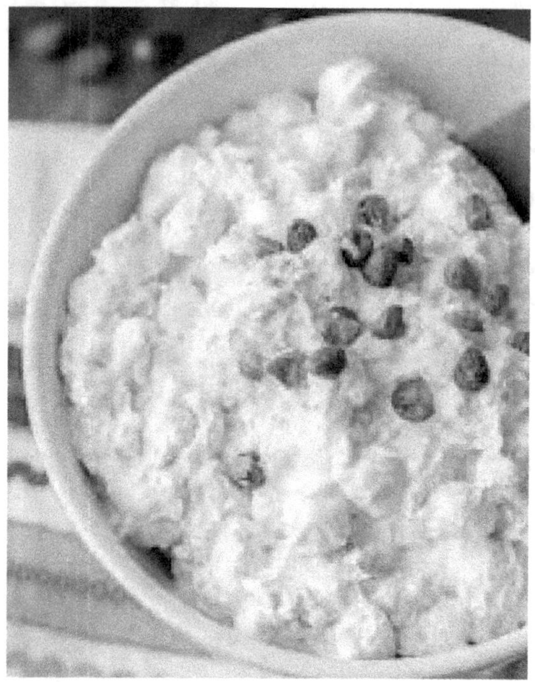

Servings: 2

Preparation Time: 10 minutes

Ingredients:

1 tablespoon olive oil

½ cup pistachios, unsalted

1 cucumber, sliced

1 ½ cups cherry tomatoes

¼ cup basil, chopped

2 cups baby salad greens

2 tablespoons sherry vinegar

Pinch of salt

Pinch of pepper

Directions:

Preheat the oven to 350°f. Grease a baking sheet with olive oil.

Spread pistachios in the baking sheet. Place inside the oven and toast for 8 minutes. Set aside.

Meanwhile, put together cucumber, tomatoes, basil, and baby salad greens. Season with vinegar, salt, and pepper. Coat well. Add the pistachios. Serve.

Nutrition:
protein 7.51g
potassium (k) 525 mg
sodium, Na 97 mg

Banana cookies

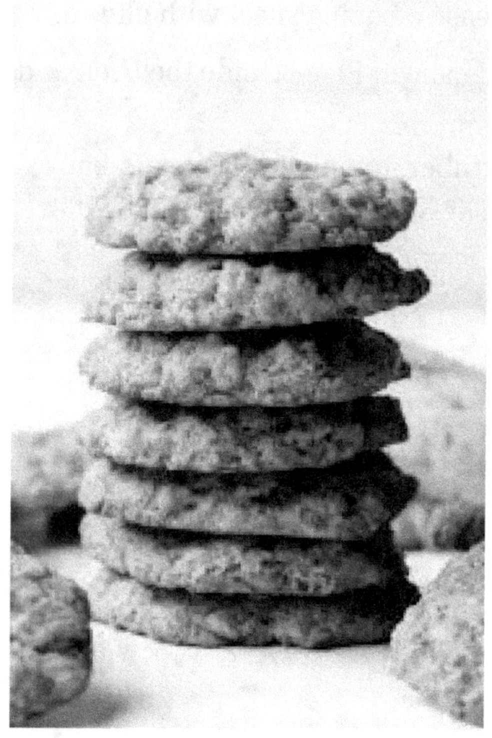

Servings: 8

Preparation Time: 30 minutes

Ingredients:

2 ripe bananas, peeled

2/3 cup applesauce, unsweetened

¼ cup almond milk, unsweetened

4 pitted dates

1 tablespoon cinnamon

2/3 cup coconut flour

1 teaspoon vanilla

1 1/2 teaspoons lemon juice

3 tablespoons dried and chopped cranberries

1 teaspoon baking powder

2 tablespoons dried and chopped raisins

Directions:

Preheat the oven to 350°f.

In a food processor, combine almond milk, applesauce, dates, and bananas. Blend until you achieve a smooth consistency.

Add in coconut flour, baking powder, cinnamon, vanilla, and lemon juice. Blend for 1 minute. Fold in cranberries and raisins.

Pour a baking sheet with the cookie dough. Place inside the oven for 20 minutes.

Allow to sit for 5 minutes and let it harden. Serve.

Nutrition:
protein 1.05g
potassium (k) 309 mg
sodium, Na 28 mg

Baked cinnamon over apple raisins

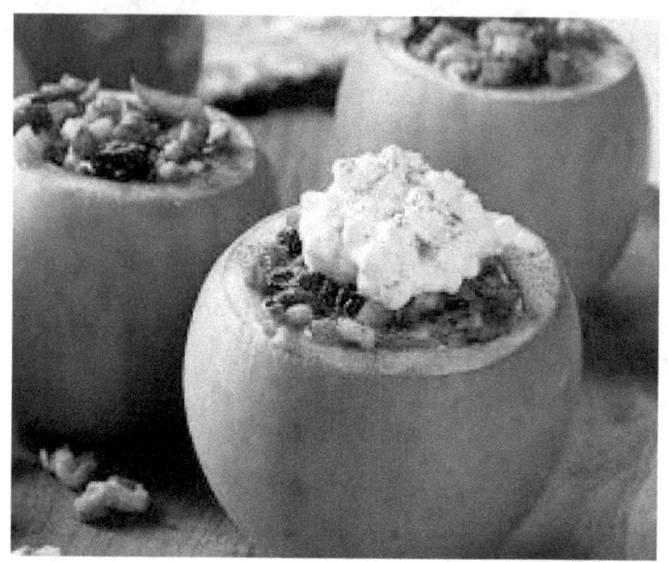

Servings: 4

Preparation Time: 10 minutes

Ingredients:

4 apples, cored

¼ cup raisins

½ cup 100% apple juice

1/8 teaspoon nutmeg

1 tablespoon lemon juice

½ teaspoon ground cinnamon

2 tablespoons brown sugar

1 teaspoon lemon peel, grated

Directions:

Layer apples in a baking dish. Fill them with raisins.

Meanwhile, in a small bowl, put together apple juice, nutmeg, lemon juice, ground cinnamon, brown sugar, and lemon peel. Mix ingredients until well-combined.

Coat apples with the mixture. Cover with plastic wrap. Set aside.

For the remaining cinnamon, place inside the microwave and heat for 4 minutes or until the sauce thickens.

Drizzle over apples. Serve.

Nutrition:
protein 0.82g
potassium (k) 303 mg
sodium, Na 5 mg

Choco berry almonds

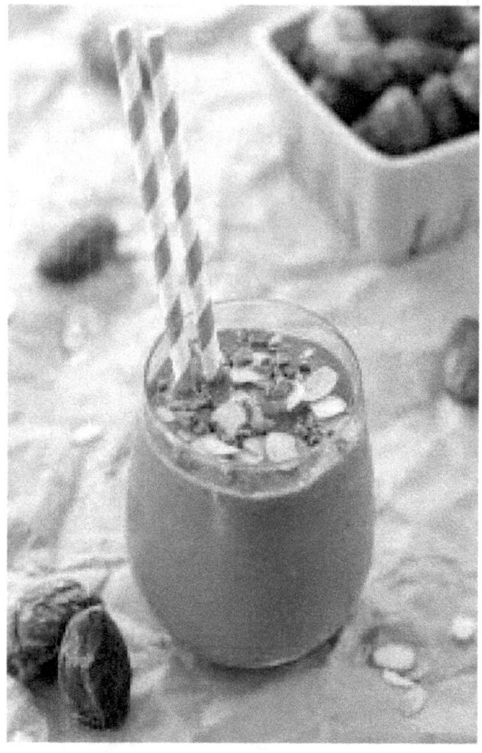

Servings: 2

Preparation Time: 1 hour

Ingredients:

½ cup dark chocolate

2 cups berries, chopped into bite-sized pieces

½ cup raw almonds, crushed

Directions:

Melt the chocolate in a microwave-safe bowl for 1 minute and 30 seconds.

Roll chopped bananas on the melted chocolate. Roll over almonds.

Refrigerate for 1 hour. Serve.

Nutrition:
protein 8.12g
potassium (k) 722 mg
sodium, Na 6 mg

Honey cinnamon bananas

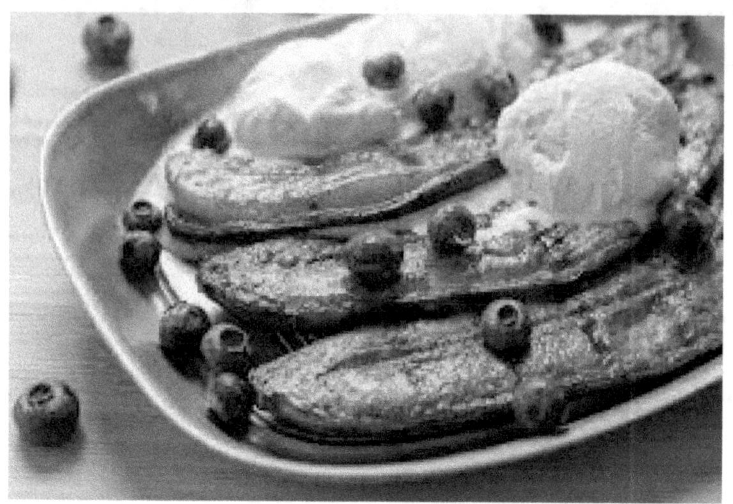

Servings: 1

Preparation Time: 5 minutes

Ingredients:

1 large banana, chopped into ½ inch pieces

2 teaspoons honey

1 teaspoon cinnamon

Directions:

In a small bowl, combine honey and cinnamon.

Heat the olive oil in a pan. Cook banana slices for 2 minutes or until browned all over.

Pour honey and cinnamon mixture over the bananas. Serve.

Nutrition:
protein 1.63g
potassium (k) 505 mg
sodium, Na 2 mg

Cinnamon apple sauté

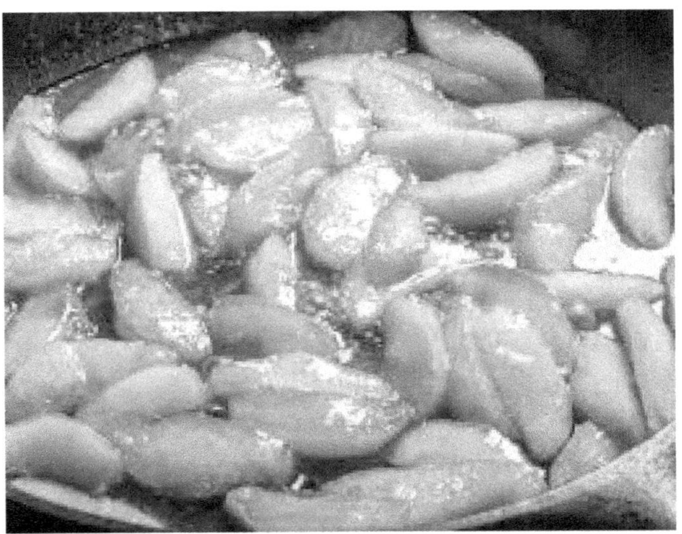

Servings: 1

Preparation Time: 5 minutes

Ingredients:

1 teaspoon cinnamon

1 apple, chopped into bite-sized pieces

½ teaspoon coconut oil

Directions:

Heat the pan. Pour coconut oil. Put the chopped apples.

Dab some cinnamon and mix well. Continue mixing for 2 minutes or until the mixture has caramelized. Serve.

Nutrition:
protein 0.69g
potassium (k) 206 mg
sodium, Na 0 mg

Gluten-free dark Choco almond butter

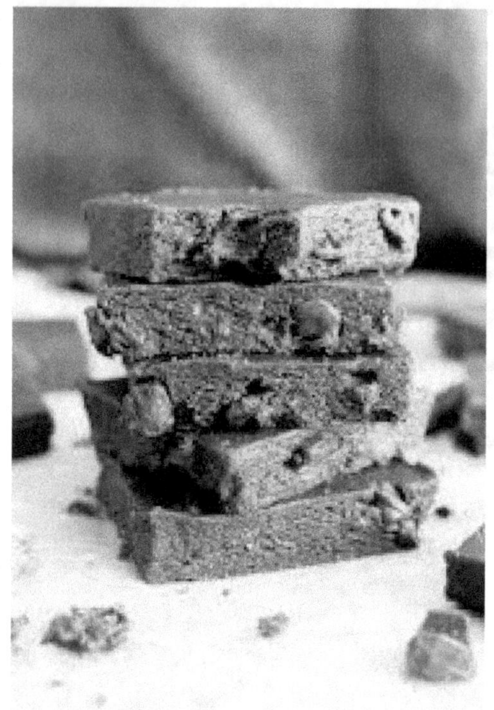

Servings: 8

Preparation Time: 20 minutes

Ingredients:

½ teaspoon baking soda

1 cup almond butter

1 egg, large

¾ cup sugar

½ teaspoon salt

½ cup dark chocolate, chopped

Directions:

Preheat the oven to 350°f. Line a baking sheet.

Meanwhile, put together baking soda, almond butter, egg, sugar, and salt. Mix until all ingredients are well-combined.

Fold in chocolate. Mix until it forms a dough.

Spoon an equal amount of mixture on a baking sheet. Place inside the oven and bake for 10 minutes.

Allow cookies to cool before serving

Nutrition:
protein 7.83g
potassium (k) 288 mg
sodium, Na 237mg

Mango pear salsa

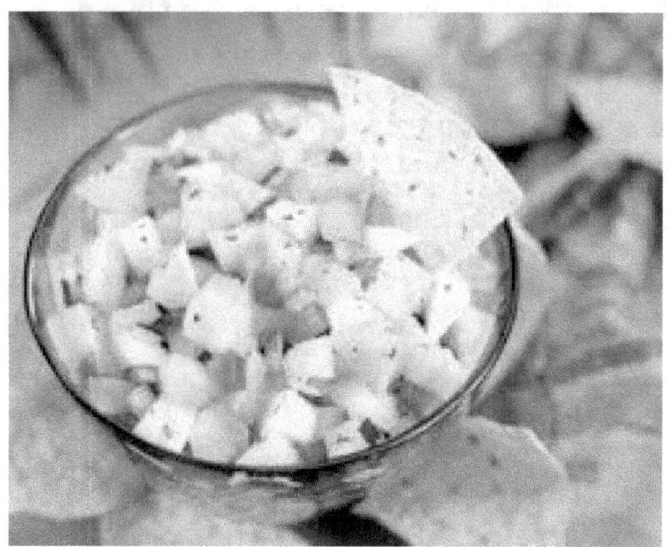

Servings: 8 (½ cup per serving)

Preparation Time: 10 minutes

Ingredients:

1 mango, chunked

¼ cup red onion, finely chopped

2 pears, cored, chunked

1/4 cup yellow bell pepper, finely chopped

1/4 cup red bell pepper, finely chopped

2 teaspoon olive oil

3 tablespoons fresh cilantro, chopped

1 jalapeño pepper, finely chopped

Pinch of salt

1 tablespoon lime juice

Directions:

Mix mango, red onion, pears, yellow bell pepper, red bell
pepper, olive oil, cilantro, jalapeño pepper, salt, and lime juice
in a bowl. Mix well until all ingredients are well combined.
Wrap bowl.

Place inside the refrigerator. Serve as needed.

Nutrition:
protein 0.77g

potassium (k) 171 mg
sodium, Na 22mg

Zucchini chips

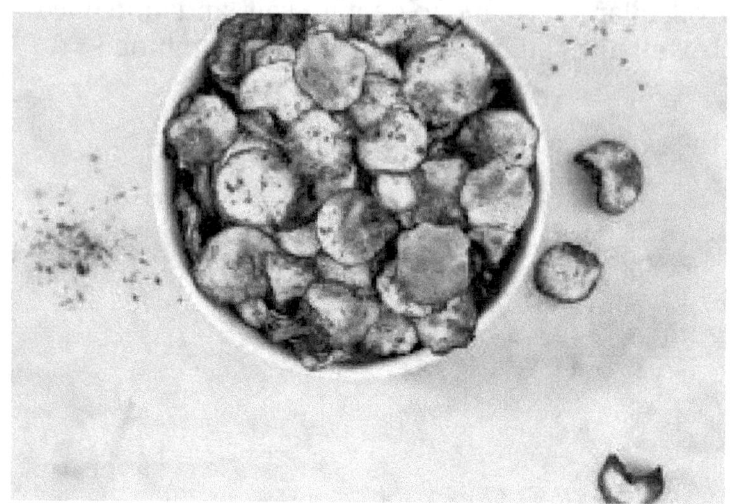

Servings: 4

Preparation Time: 2 hours

Ingredients:

4 zucchinis, sliced thinly, ends removed

2 tablespoons apple cider vinegar

2 tablespoons olive oil

¼ teaspoon salt

¼ teaspoon ground black pepper

Directions:

Preheat the oven to 225°f. Line a baking dish with parchment paper.

In a small bowl, pour vinegar, oil, salt, and pepper. Add zucchini. Mix all ingredients until the zucchini slices are well coated.

Layer coated zucchini in baking sheets. Place inside the oven. Bake for 2 hours.

Remove zucchini chips and let cool. Serve as needed. Leftovers can be stored in an airtight container.

Nutrition:

protein 2.39g
potassium (k) 519 mg

sodium 162 mg

Lunch recipes

Mexican beef flour wrap

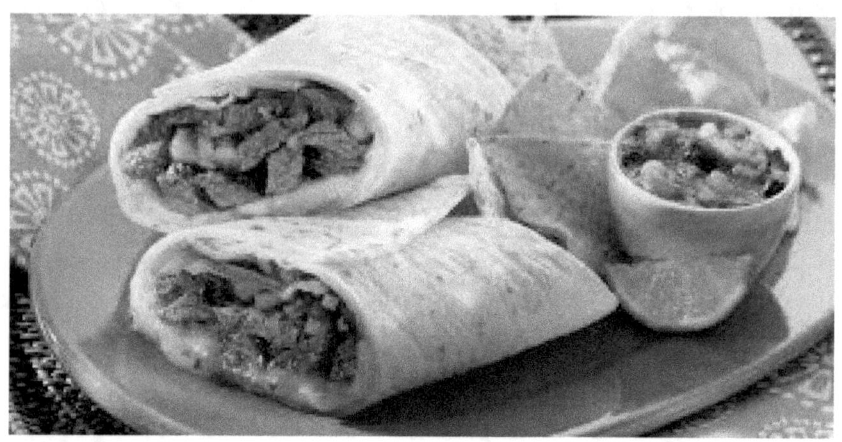

Servings: 2

Preparation Time: 10 minutes

Ingredients:

5 oz. Cooked roast beef

8 cucumber slices

2 flour tortillas, 6-inch size

2 tbsp. Whipped cream cheese

2 leaves light green lettuce

1/4 bowl cut red onion

1/4 stripped cut sweet bell pepper

1 tsp. Herb seasoning blend

Directions:

Spread the cheese over the flour wraps. Try to use the ingredients to make two wraps.

Layer the tortillas with roast beef, onions, lettuce, pepper strips and cucumber.

Sprinkle with the herb seasoning

Roll up the wraps and cut them into 4 pieces each. Serve fresh. Enjoy!

Nutrition:

Calories: 255

Protein: 24 g

Sodium: 275 mg

Potassium: 445 mg

Phosphorus: 250 mg

Mixed chorizo in egg flour wraps

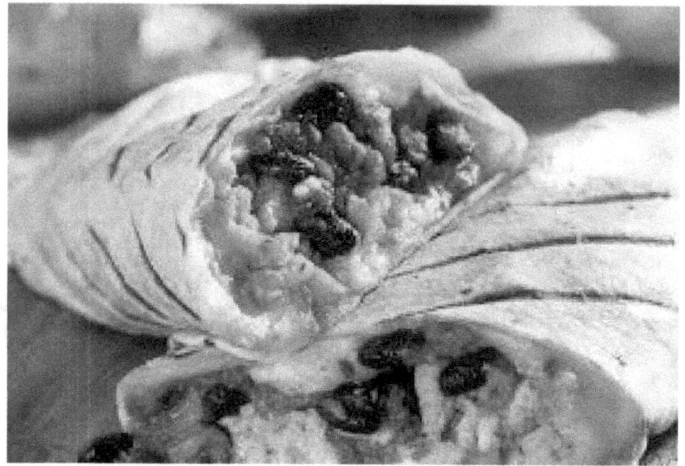

Servings: 2

Preparation Time: 10 minutes

Ingredients:

1 pack chorizo

1 egg

1 flour tortilla or 6-inch size

Direction

Cook the chorizo in a pan on stove, cutting the meat into small pieces.

Eliminate excessive water or fat and add 1 egg combining all while they are being cooked.

Serve everything on a flour tortilla or wrapping the tortillas. Enjoy!

Nutrition:

Calories: 223

Protein: 15 g

Sodium: 315 mg

Potassium: 285 mg

Phosphorus: 230 mg

Sandwich with chicken salad

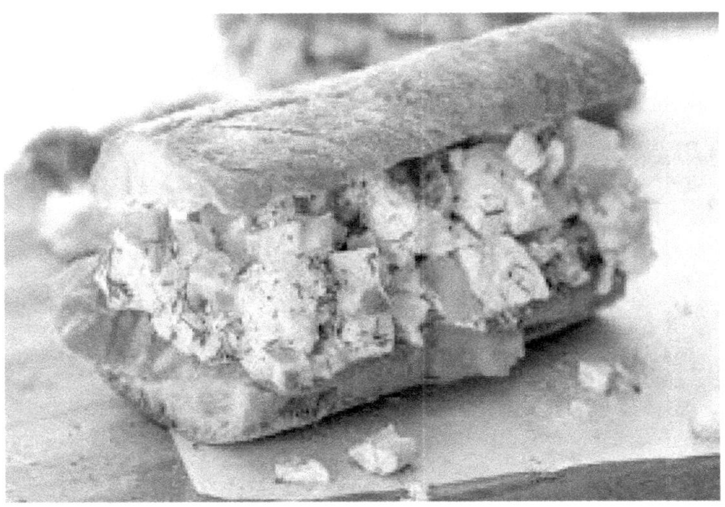

Servings: 2

Preparation Time: 10 minutes

Ingredients:

2 bowls cooked chicken

1/2 cup low-fat mayonnaise

1/2 cup green bell pepper

1 cup pieces pineapple

1/3 cup carrots

4 slices flatbread

1/2 tsp. Black pepper

Directions:

Prepare aside the diced chicken and drain pineapple, adding green bell pepper, black pepper and carrots.

Combine all in a bowl and refrigerate until chilled.

Later on, serve the chicken salad on the flatbread. Enjoy!

Nutrition:

Calories: 345

Protein: 22 g

Sodium: 395 mg

Potassium: 330 mg

Phosphorus: 165 mg

Spice bread with tuna salad

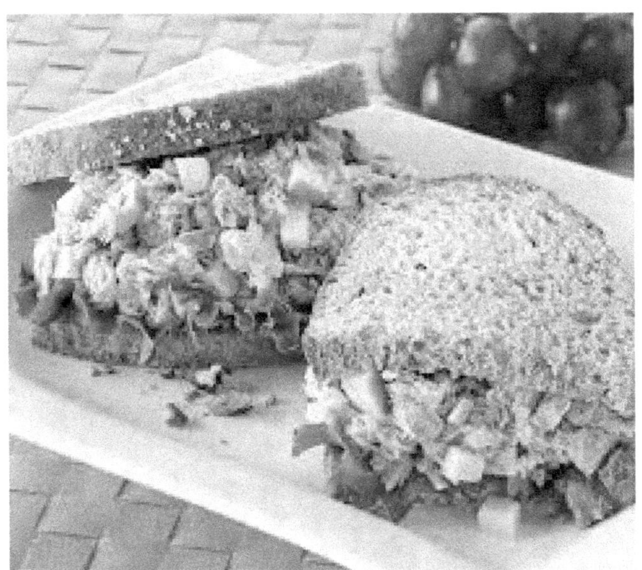

Servings: 2

Preparation Time: 10 minutes

Ingredients:

1 tbsp. Onion

1-piece celery

1 fresh tomato

Some lettuce leaves

1 tbsp. Low calories mayonnaise

1 medium bagel or spiced bread

1/2 pack low sodium water-packed canned tuna

Directions:

Chop onion, tomato and celery.

Open tuna and cut into small pieces.

Put everything in the bagel on the lettuce leaves, adding some mayonnaise and then close the bread. Serve and enjoy!

Nutrition:

Calories: 290

Protein: 25 g

Sodium: 475 mg

Potassium: 320 mg

Phosphorus: 175 mg

Tiny rice pies

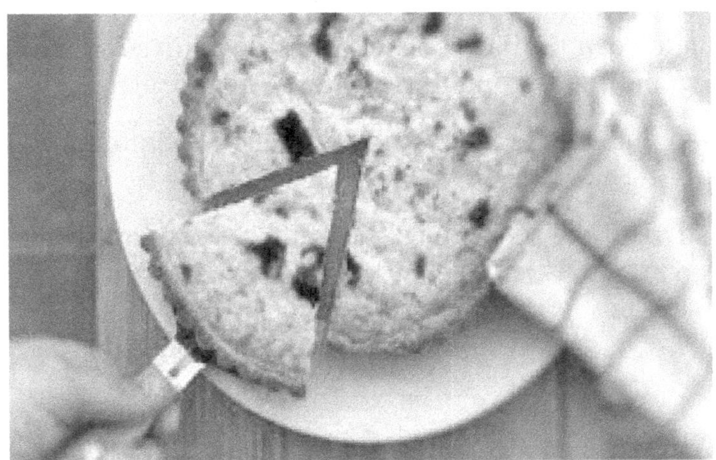

Servings: 2

Preparation Time: 10 minutes

Ingredients:

2 tbsp. Vegetable oil

1 tsp. Mustard seeds

1/2 cup semolina

2 green finely cut chilies

1/8 tsp. Salt

1/4 cup yogurt

1/4 glass water

1/4 grated corn

1/4 Indian cheese

Some bits finely cut cilantro

1 tbsp. Clarified butter

Directions:

Heat the oil and the seeds in a pan and add semolina, chilies and a bit of salt.

Cook it until the semolina becomes a bit brown. Let it cool down. Put together yogurt with some water and mix it until it is smooth, then add corn, Indian cheese, cilantro, yogurt and add everything to semolina, leaving it aside for 10-15 minutes.

Put the clarified butter in a pan, steaming then the semolina mix for 10 minutes.

Put some cilantro on the semolina circles and serve them still a bit warm. Enjoy!

Nutrition:

Calories: 175

Protein: 5 g

Sodium: 214 mg

Potassium: 140 mg

Phosphorus: 89 mg

Toast topped with creamy eggs

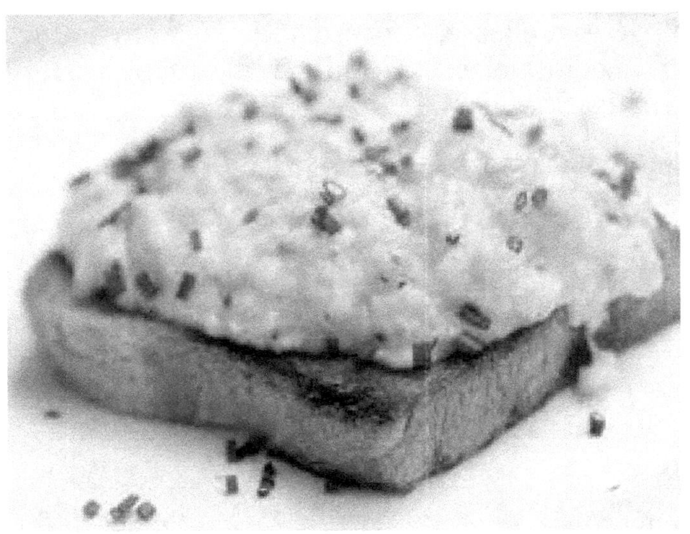

Servings: 2

Preparation Time: 15 minutes

Ingredients:

4 slices white bread

6 eggs

4 oz. Cream cheese

3 tbsp. Unsalted butter

1/3 cup flour

1 1/2 cups unsweetened, plain almond milk

1/2 tbsp. Yellow mustard

1/8 tsp. Pepper

Directions:

Hard boil the eggs for 12 minutes. Remove them from heat, drain and cover with cool water.

Peel and chop boiled eggs. Put together the butter and flour in a sauce pan at medium low heat.

Mix constantly until well combined.

Add almond milk, cream cheese, mustard and pepper to butter and flour mixture. Let it thicken and add the eggs to the sauce, keeping at a warm heat.

Toast the bread and put the egg mixture over the toast before serving
Enjoy!

Nutrition:

Calories: 430

Protein: 15 g

Sodium: 400 mg

Potassium: 250 mg

Phosphorus: 210 mg

Fresh cucumber soup

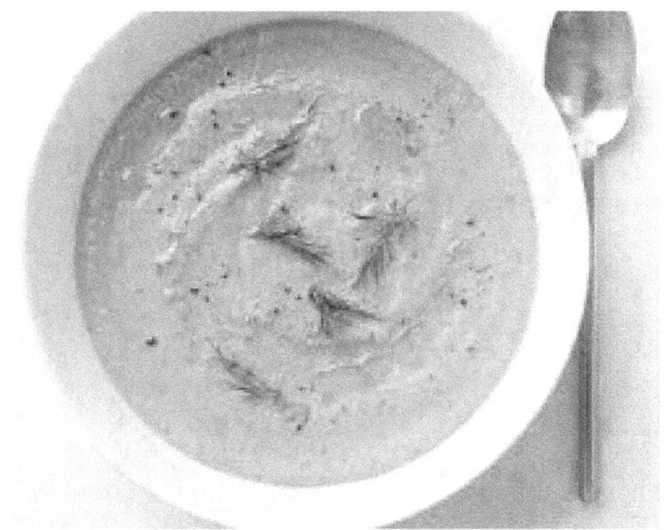

Servings: 2

Preparation Time: 2 hours 5 minutes

Ingredients:

2 cucumbers

1/3 cup white onion

1 green onion

1/4 cup fresh mint

2 tbsp. Fresh lemon juice

2 tbsp. Fresh dill

2/3 cup water

1/3 cup sour cream

1/2 cup half and half cream

1/2 tsp. Pepper

1/4 tsp. Salt

Directions:

Remove both peel and seeds from cucumbers.

Cut mint and the onions. Cut up dill.

Put all ingredients in a mixer and whisk until smooth.

Cover and place in the refrigerator for at least 2 hours.

Use fresh dill sprigs to garnish the soup. Serve and enjoy!

Nutrition:

Calories: 78

Protein: 2 g

Sodium: 127 mg

Potassium: 257 mg

Phosphorus: 65 mg

Berry salad with Italian ricotta cheese

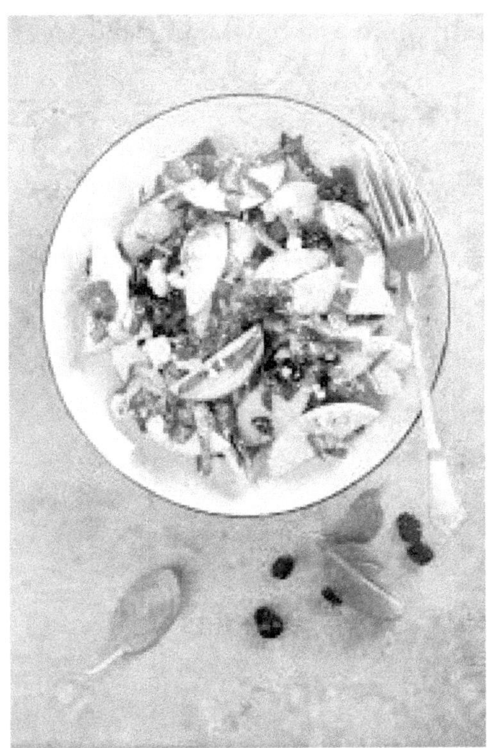

Servings: 2

Preparation Time: 5 minutes

Ingredients:

1 cup fresh blackberries

1 cup fresh blueberries

2 cups fresh strawberries

1/3 cup lemon juice

2 cups fresh Italian ricotta cheese

1/8 tsp. Cinnamon

Directions:

Wash well both blackberries and blueberries and strawberries. Slice them and put them all together.

Add some lemon juice from the cup.

Put the ricotta cheese on a round plate or a bowl and then cover it with berries.

Spread the cinnamon on it. Serve and enjoy!

Nutrition:

Calories: 140

Protein: 15 g

Sodium: 380 mg

Potassium: 350 mg

Phosphorus: 180 mg

Celery tuna salad

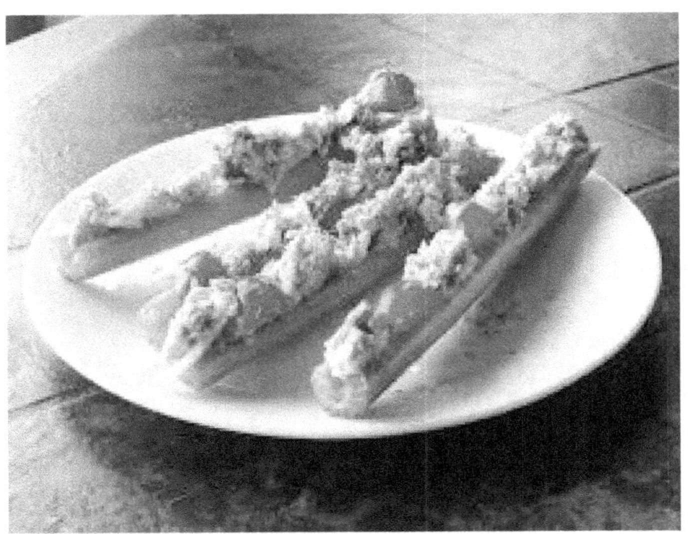

Servings: 2

Preparation Time: 5 minutes

Ingredients:

1-piece celery

15 oz. Packed and unsalted tuna

1/2 apple

1/2 small onion

2 tbsp. Mayonnaise

A bit of black pepper

Pinch salt

Directions:

Prepare the tuna and cut the apple, celery and onion.

Mix all together, adding mayonnaise, black pepper and if you wish, some salt.

Serve on lettuce and with unsalted crackers. Enjoy!

Nutrition:

Calories: 20

Protein: 15 g

Sodium: 185 mg

Potassium: 318 mg

Phosphorus: 183 mg

Meat casserole

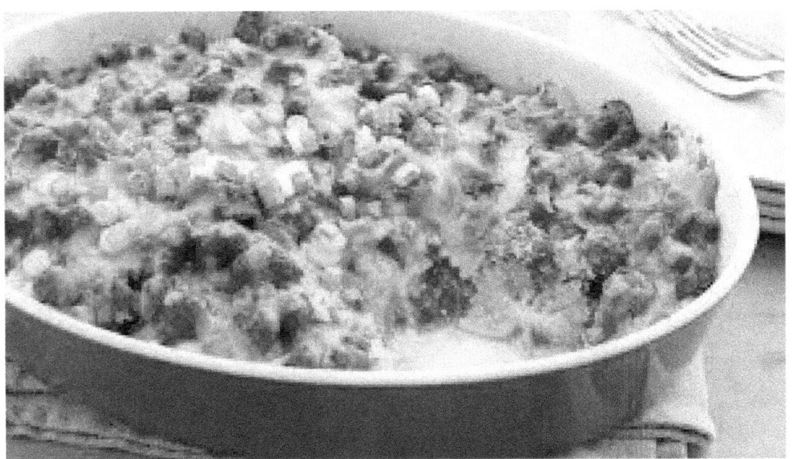

Servings: 2

Preparation Time: 60 minutes

Ingredients:

10 oz. Reduced-fat pork sausage

8 oz. Cream cheese

1 glass low-fat milk

4 slices white bread

5 eggs

1/2 tsp. Dry mustard

1/2 dry onion flakes

Directions:

Preheat oven at 325°f (160°c).

Cut the sausage and cook in a cooking dish. Set aside and mix all other ingredients.

Add cooked sausage to mixture and place bread pieces in a square casserole, pour sausage mix over the bread and cook for 50 minutes.

Cut into 10 portions and serve. Enjoy!

Nutrition:

Calories: 222

Protein: 10 g

Sodium: 355 mg

Potassium: 200 mg

Phosphorus: 156 mg

Ground beef in a cup

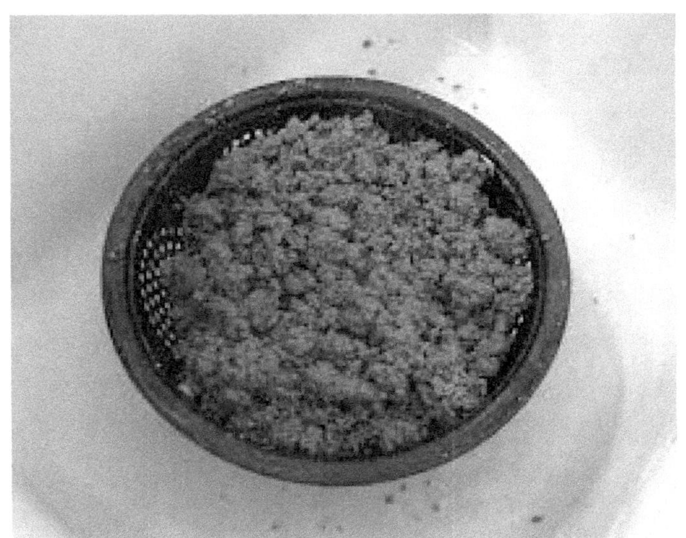

Servings: 2

Preparation Time: 10 minutes

Ingredients:

1/4-pound ground beef

2 tbsp. Low fat milk

2 tsp. Ketchup

2 tbsp. Quick-cooked oats

1 tsp. Onion powder

Directions:

Spray a large cup with non-stick cooking spray.

In another cup put together the milk (or its substitute), ketchup, onion, oats.

Crumble meat over the mixture and mix everything, pressing the ground beef.

Cover and put it in the microwave for 3 minutes (high) and serve it very warm. Enjoy!

Nutrition:

Calories: 250

Protein: 25 g

Sodium: 160 mg

Potassium: 395 mg

Phosphorus: 245 mg

Dinner recipes

Eggplant and red pepper soup

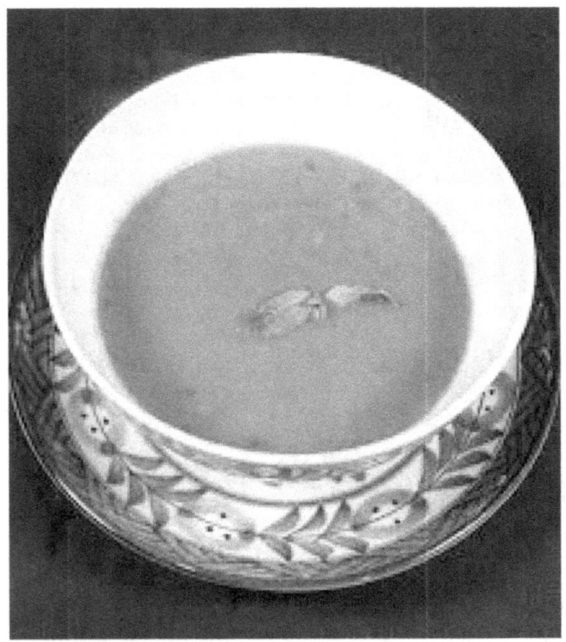

Preparation time: 20 minutes
cooking time: 40 minutes
servings: 6

Ingredients

Sweet onion – 1 small, cut into quarters

Small red bell peppers – 2, halved

Cubed eggplant – 2 cups

Garlic – 2 cloves, crushed

Olive oil – 1 tbsp.

Chicken stock – 1 cup

Water

Chopped fresh basil – ¼ cup

Ground black pepper

Directions:

Preheat the oven to 350f.

Put the onions, red peppers, eggplant, and garlic in a baking dish.

Drizzle the vegetables with the olive oil.

Roast the vegetables for 30 minutes or until they are slightly charred and soft.

Cool the vegetables slightly and remove the skin from the peppers.

Puree the vegetables with a hand mixer (with the chicken stock).

Transfer the soup to a medium pot and add enough water to reach the desired thickness.

Heat the soup to a simmer and add the basil.

Season with pepper and serve.

Nutrition:

Calories: 61

Fat: 2g

Carb: 9g

Phosphorus: 33mg

Potassium: 198mg

Sodium: 98mg

Protein: 2g

Seafood casserole

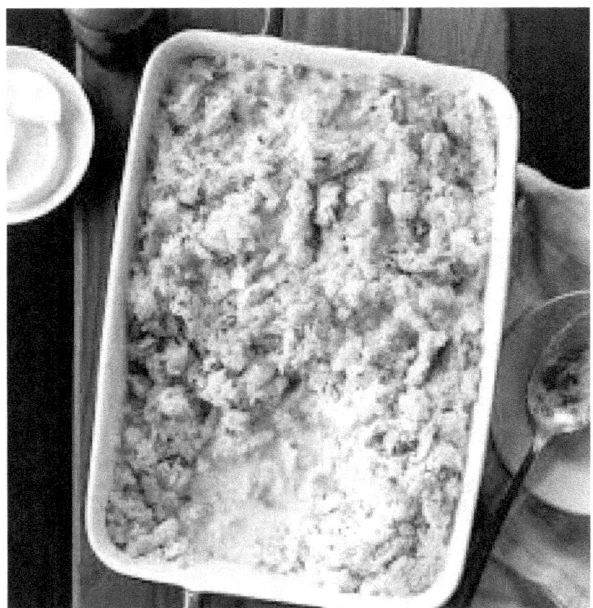

Preparation time: 20 minutes
cooking time: 45 minutes
servings: 6

Ingredients

Eggplant – 2 cups, peeled and diced into 1-inch pieces

Butter, for greasing the baking dish

Olive oil – 1 tbsp.

Sweet onion – ½, chopped

Minced garlic - 1 tsp.

Celery stalk – 1, chopped

Red bell pepper – ½, boiled and chopped

Freshly squeezed lemon juice – 3 tbsps.

Hot sauce – 1 tsp.

Creole seasoning mix – ¼ tsp.

White rice – ½ cup, uncooked

Egg – 1 large

Cooked shrimp – 4 ounces

Queen crab meat – 6 ounces

Directions:

Preheat the oven to 350f.

Boil the eggplant in a saucepan for 5 minutes. Drain and set aside.

Grease a 9-by-13-inch baking dish with butter and set aside.

Heat the olive oil in a large skillet over medium heat.

Sauté the garlic, onion, celery, and bell pepper for 4 minutes or until tender.

Add the sautéed vegetables to the eggplant, along with the lemon juice, hot sauce, seasoning, rice, and egg

Stir to combine.

Fold in the shrimp and crab meat.

Spoon the casserole mixture into the casserole dish, patting down the top.

1 Bake for 25 to 30 minutes or until casserole is heated through and rice is tender.

1 Serve warm.

Nutrition:

Calories: 118

Fat: 4g

Carb: 9g

Phosphorus: 102mg

Potassium: 199mg

Sodium: 235mg

Protein: 12g

Ground beef and rice soup

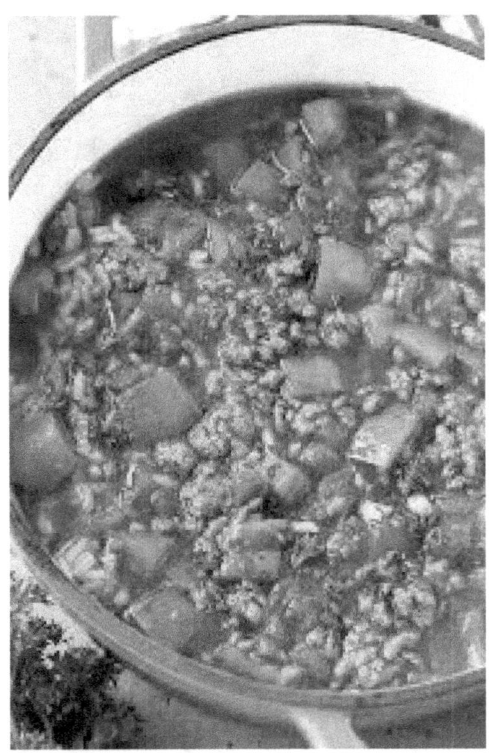

Preparation time: 15 minutes
cooking time: 40 minutes
servings: 6

Ingredients

Extra-lean ground beef – ½ pound

Small sweet onion – ½, chopped

Minced garlic – 1 tsp.

Water – 2 cups

Low-sodium beef broth – 1 cup

Long-grain white rice – ½ cup, uncooked

Celery stalk – 1, chopped

Fresh green beans – ½ cup, cut into – 1-inch pieces

Chopped fresh thyme – 1 tsp.

Ground black pepper

Directions:

Sauté the ground beef in a saucepan for 6 minutes or until the beef is completely browned.

Drain off the excess fat and add the onion and garlic to the saucepan.

Sauté the vegetables for about 3 minutes, or until they are softened.

Add the celery, rice, beef broth, and water.

Bring the soup to a boil, reduce the heat to low and simmer for 30 minutes or until the rice is tender.

Add the green beans and thyme and simmer for 3 minutes.

Remove the soup from the heat and season with pepper.

Nutrition:

Calories: 154

Fat: 7g

Carb: 14g

Phosphorus: 76mg

Potassium: 179mg

Sodium: 133mg

Protein: 9g

Couscous burgers

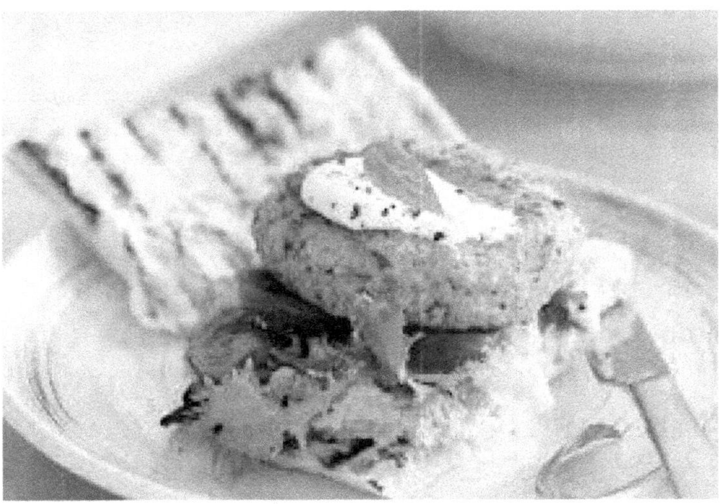

Preparation time: 20 minutes
cooking time: 10 minutes
servings: 4

Ingredients

Canned chickpeas – ½ cup, rinsed and drained

Chopped fresh cilantro – 2 tbsps.

Chopped fresh parsley

Lemon juice - 1 tbsp.

Lemon zest – 2 tsps.

Minced garlic – 1 tsp.

Cooked couscous – 2 ½ cups

Eggs – 2 lightly beaten

Olive oil – 2 tbsps.

Directions:

Put the cilantro, chickpeas, parsley, lemon juice, lemon zest, and garlic in a food processor and pulse until a paste form.

Transfer the chickpea mixture to a bowl and add the eggs and couscous. Mix well.

Chill the mixture in the refrigerator for 1 hour.

Form the couscous mixture into 4 patties.

Heat olive oil in a skillet.

Place the patties in the skillet, 2 at a time, gently pressing them down with a spatula.

Cook for 5 minutes or until golden and flip the patties over.

Cook the other side for 5 minutes and transfer the cooked burgers to a plate covered with a paper towel.

Repeat with the remaining 2 burgers.

Nutrition:

Calories: 242

Fat: 10g

Carb: 29g

Phosphorus: 108mg

Potassium: 168mg

Sodium: 43mg

Protein: 9g

Baked flounder

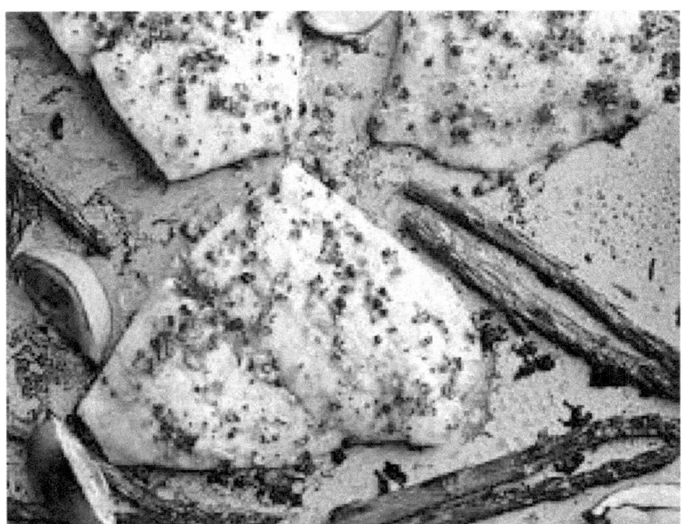

Preparation time: 20 minutes
cooking time: 5 minutes
servings: 4

Ingredients

Homemade mayonnaise – ¼ cup

Juice of 1 lime

Zest of 1 lime

Chopped fresh cilantro – ½ cup

Flounder fillets – 4 (3-ounce)

Ground black pepper

Directions:

Preheat the oven to 400f.

In a bowl, stir together the cilantro, lime juice, lime zest, and mayonnaise.

Place 4 pieces of foil, about 8 by 8 inches square, on a clean work surface.

Place a flounder fillet in the center of each square.

Top the fillets evenly with the mayonnaise mixture.

Season the flounder with pepper.

Fold the sides of the foil over the fish, creating a snug packet, and place the foil packets on a baking sheet.

Bake the fish for 4 to 5 minutes.

Unfold the packets and serve.

Nutrition:

Calories: 92

Fat: 4g

Carb: 2g

Phosphorus: 208mg

Potassium: 137mg

Sodium: 267mg

Protein: 12g

Persian chicken

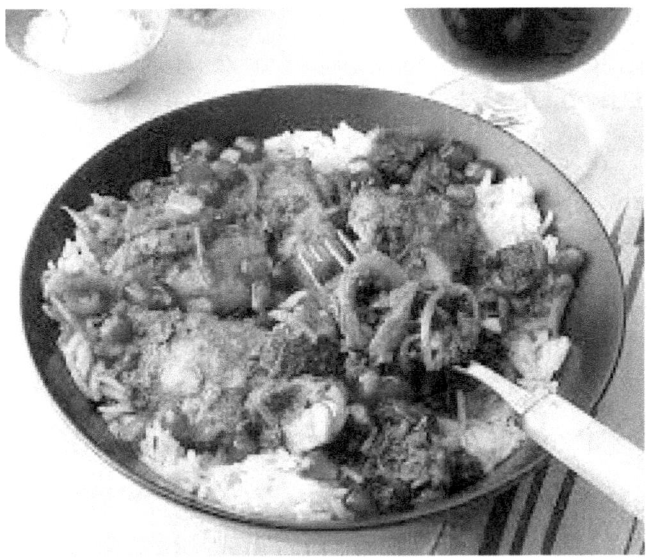

Preparation time: 10 minutes
cooking time: 20 minutes
servings: 5

Ingredients

Sweet onion – ½, chopped

Lemon juice – ¼ cup

Dried oregano – 1 tbsp.

Minced garlic – 1 tsp.

Sweet paprika – 1 tsp.

Ground cumin – ½ tsp.

Olive oil – ½ cup

Boneless, skinless chicken thighs – 5

Directions:

Put the cumin, paprika, garlic, oregano, lemon juice, and onion in a food processor and pulse to mix the ingredients.

Keep the motor running and add the olive oil until the mixture is smooth.

Place the chicken thighs in a large sealable freezer bag and pour the marinade into the bag

Seal the bag and place in the refrigerator, turning the bag twice, for 2 hours.

Remove the thighs from the marinade and discard the extra marinade.

Preheat the barbecue to medium.

Grill the chicken for about 20 minutes, turning once, until it reaches 165f.

Nutrition:

Calories: 321

Fat: 21g

Carb: 3g

Phosphorus: 131mg

Potassium: 220mg

Sodium: 86mg

Protein: 22g

Pork souvlaki

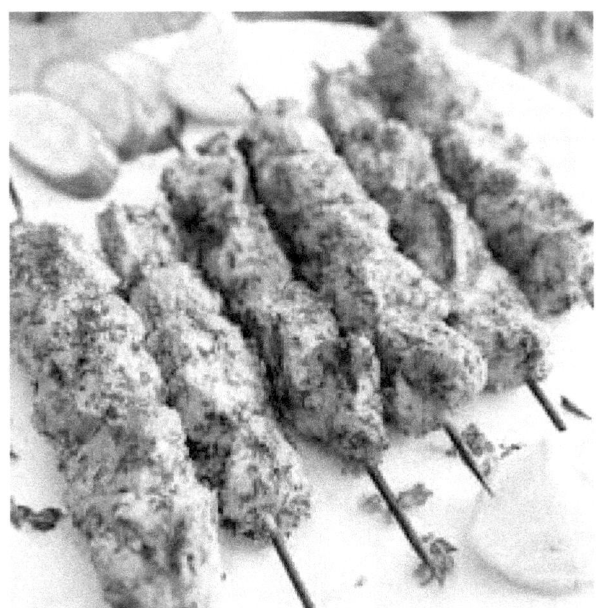

Preparation time: 20 minutes
cooking time: 12 minutes
servings: 8

Ingredients

Olive oil – 3 tbsps.

Lemon juice – 2 tbsps.

Minced garlic – 1 tsp.

Chopped fresh oregano – 1 tbsp.

Ground black pepper – ¼ tsp.

Pork leg – 1 pound, cut in 2-inch cubes

Directions:

In a bowl, stir together the lemon juice, olive oil, garlic, oregano, and pepper.

Add the pork cubes and toss to coat.

Place the bowl in the refrigerator, covered, for 2 hours to marinate.

Thread the pork chunks onto 8 wooden skewers that have been soaked in water.

Preheat the barbecue to medium-high heat.

Grill the pork skewers for about 12 minutes, turning once, until just cooked through but still juicy.

Nutrition:

Calories: 95

Fat: 4g

Carb: 0g

Phosphorus: 125mg

Potassium: 230mg

Sodium: 29mg

Protein: 13g

Pork meatloaf

Preparation time: 10 minutes
cooking time: 50 minutes
servings: 8

Ingredients

95% lean ground beef – 1 pound

Breadcrumbs – ½ cup

Chopped sweet onion – ½ cup

Egg – 1

Chopped fresh basil – 2 tbsps.

Chopped fresh thyme -1 tsp.

Chopped fresh parsley – 1 tsp.

Ground black pepper – ¼ tsp.

Brown sugar – 1 tbsp.

White vinegar – 1 tsp.

Garlic powder – ¼ tsp.

Directions:

Preheat the oven to 350f.

Mix together the breadcrumbs, beef, onion, basil, egg, thyme, parsley, and pepper until well combined.

Press the meat mixture into a 9-by-5-inch loaf pan.

In a small bowl, stir together the brown sugar, vinegar, and garlic powder.

Spread the brown sugar mixture evenly over the meat.

Bake the meatloaf for about 50 minutes or until it is cooked through.

Let the meatloaf stand for 10 minutes and then pour out any accumulated grease.

Nutrition:

Calories: 103

Fat: 3g

Carb: 7g

Phosphorus: 112mg

Potassium: 190mg

Sodium: 87mg

Protein: 11g

Chicken stew

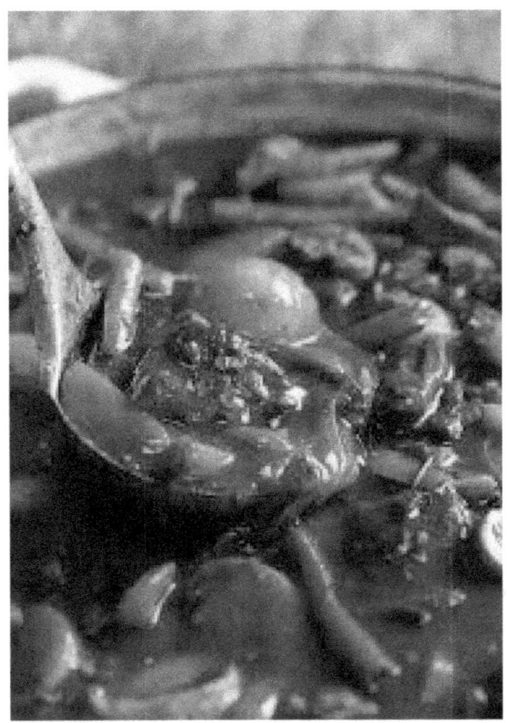

Preparation time: 20 minutes
cooking time: 50 minutes
servings: 6

Ingredients

Olive oil – 1 tbsp.

Boneless, skinless chicken thighs – 1 pound, cut into 1-inch
cubes

Sweet onion – ½, chopped

Minced garlic – 1 tbsp.

Chicken stock – 2 cups

Water – 1 cup, plus 2 tbsps.

Carrot – 1, sliced

Celery – 2 stalks, sliced

Turnip – 1, sliced thin

Chopped fresh thyme – 1 tbsp.

Chopped fresh rosemary – 1 tsp.

Cornstarch – 2 tsps.

Ground black pepper to taste

Directions:

Place a large saucepan on medium heat and add the olive oil.

Sauté the chicken for 6 minutes or until it is lightly browned, stirring often.

Add the onion and garlic, and sauté for 3 minutes.

Add 1-cup water, chicken stock, carrot, celery, and turnip and bring the stew to a boil.

Reduce the heat to low and simmer for 30 minutes or until the chicken is cooked through and tender.

Add the thyme and rosemary and simmer for 3 minutes more.

In a small bowl, stir together the 2 tbsps. Of water and the cornstarch
add the mixture to the stew.

Stir to incorporate the cornstarch mixture and cook for 3 to 4 minutes or until the stew thickens.

Remove from the heat and season with pepper.

Nutrition:

Calories: 141

Fat: 8g

Carb: 5g

Phosphorus: 53mg

Potassium: 192mg

Sodium: 214mg

Protein: 9g

Beef chili

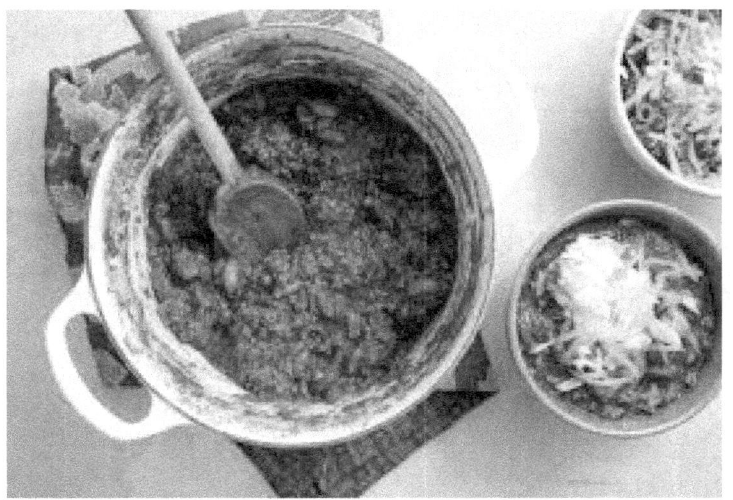

Preparation time: 10 minutes
cooking time: 30 minutes
servings: 2

Ingredients

Onion – 1, diced

Red bell pepper – 1, diced

Garlic – 2 cloves, minced

Lean ground beef – 6 oz.

Chili powder – 1 tsp.

Oregano – 1 tsp.

Extra virgin olive oil – 2 tbsps.

Water – 1 cup

Brown rice -1 cup

Fresh cilantro – 1 tbsp. To serve

Directions:

Soak vegetables in warm water.

Bring a pan of water to the boil and add rice for 20 minutes.

Meanwhile, add the oil to a pan and heat on medium-high heat.

Add the pepper, onions, and garlic and sauté for 5 minutes until soft.

Remove and set aside.

Add the beef to the pan and stir until browned.

Add the vegetables back into the pan and stir.

Now add the chili powder and herbs and the water, cover and turn the heat down a little to simmer for 15 minutes.

Meanwhile, drain the water from the rice, and the lid and steam while the chili is cooking

Serve hot with the fresh cilantro sprinkled over the top.

Nutrition:

Calories: 459

Fat: 22g

Carb: 36g

Phosphorus: 332mg

Potassium: 360mg

Sodium: 33mg

Protein: 22g

Poultry and meat mains

Baked pork chops

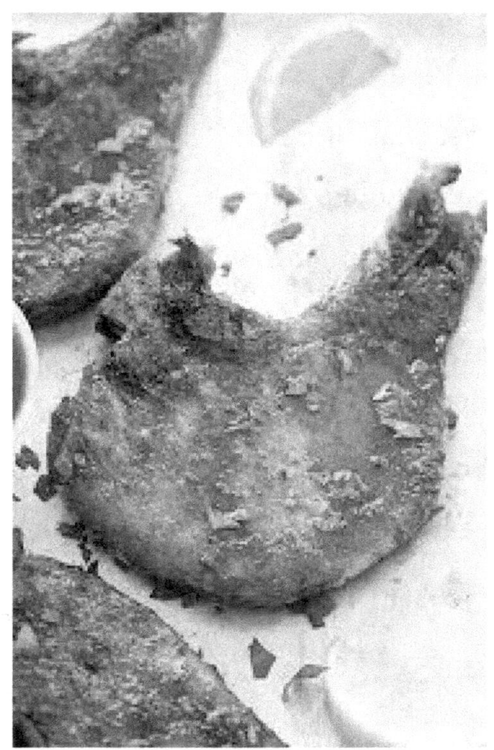

Preparation time: 10 minutes

Cooking time: 40 minutes

Servings: 6

Ingredients:

1/2 cup all-purpose flour

1 large egg

1/4 cup water

3/4 cup cornflake crumbs

6 (3 1/2 oz) center-cut pork chops

2 tbsp unsalted margarine

1 tsp paprika

Directions:

Preheat oven to 350 degrees f.

Mix and spread flour in a shallow plate.

Whisk egg with water in another shallow bowl.

Spread the cornflakes crumbs in another plate.

Coat the pork with flour then dip in the egg mix and then in the crumbs.

Grease a baking sheet and place the chops in it.

Sprinkle the paprika on top and bake for 40 minutes.

Serve fresh.

Nutrition:
calories 282
Protein 23 g
Carbohydrates 25 g
Fat 10 g
Cholesterol 95 mg
Sodium 263 mg
Potassium 394 mg
Phosphorus 203 mg
Calcium 28 mg
Fiber 1.4 g

California pork chops

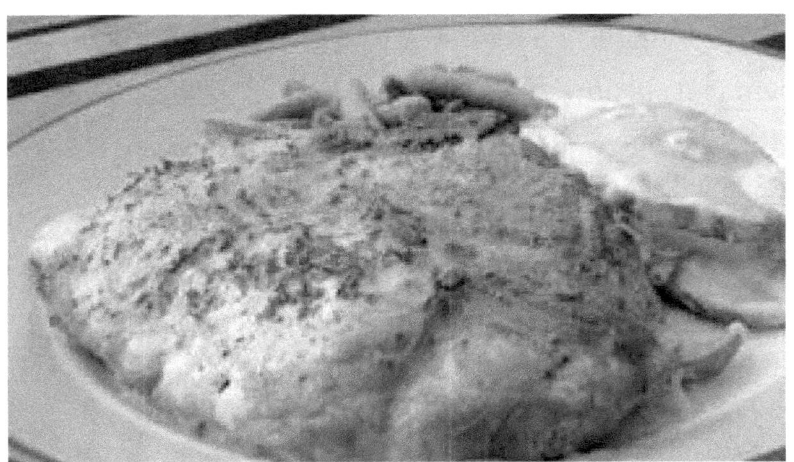

Preparation time: 10 minutes

Cooking time: 10 minutes

Servings: 2

Ingredients:

1 tbsp fresh cilantro, chopped

1/2 cup chives, chopped

2 large green bell peppers, chopped

1 lb. 1" thick boneless pork chops

1 tbsp fresh lime juice

2 cups cooked rice

1/8 tsp dried oregano leaves

1/4 tsp ground black pepper

1/4 tsp ground cumin

1 tbsp butter

1 lime

Directions:

Start by seasoning the pork chops with lime juice and cilantro.

Place them in a shallow dish.

Toss the chives with pepper, cumin, butter, oregano and rice in a bowl.

Stuff the bell peppers with this mixture and place them around the pork chops.

Cover the chop and bell peppers with a foil sheet and bake them for 10 minutes in the oven at 375 degrees f.

Serve warm.

Nutrition:
calories 265
Protein 34 g
Carbohydrates 24 g
Fat 15 g
Cholesterol 86 mg
Sodium 70 mg
Potassium 564 mg
Phosphorus 240 mg
Calcium 22 mg
Fiber 1.0 g

Beef chorizo

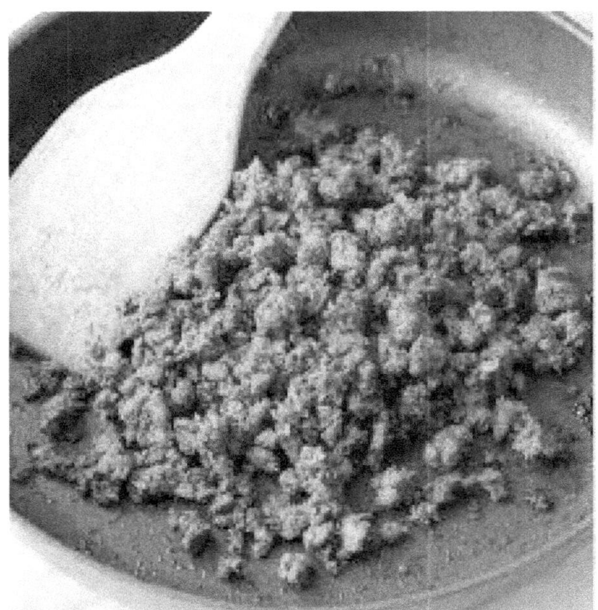

Preparation time: 10 minutes

Cooking time: 10 minutes

Servings: 4

Ingredients:

3 garlic cloves, minced

1 lb. 90% lean ground beef

2 tbsp hot chili powder

2 tsp red or cayenne pepper

1 tsp black pepper

1 tsp ground oregano

2 tsp white vinegar

Directions:

Mix all ingredients together in a bowl thoroughly then spread the mixture in a baking pan.

Bake the meat for 10 minutes at 325 degrees f in an oven.

Slice and serve in crumbles.

Nutrition:
calories 72
Protein 8 g
Carbohydrates 1 g
Fat 4 g
Cholesterol 25 mg
Sodium 46 mg
Potassium 174 mg
Phosphorus 79 mg
Calcium 14 mg
Fiber 0.8 g

Pork fajitas

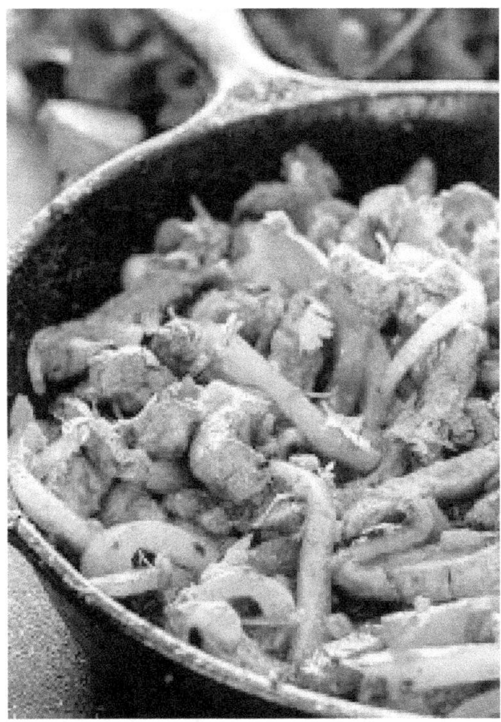

Preparation time: 10 minutes

Cooking time: 20 minutes

Servings: 4

Ingredients:

1 green bell pepper, julienned

1 medium onion, julienned

2 garlic cloves, minced

1 lb. lean, boneless pork cut into strips

1 tsp dried oregano

1/2 tsp cumin

2 tbsp pineapple juice

2 tbsp vinegar

1/4 tsp hot pepper sauce

1 tbsp canola oil

4 flour tortillas, 8" size

Directions:

Start by mixing the oregano, garlic, vinegar, cumin, hot sauce, and pineapple juice in a bowl.

Place the pork in this marinade and mix well to coat them then refrigerate for 15 minutes.

Meanwhile, preheat the oven to 325 degrees f.

Wrap the tortillas in a foil and heat them in the oven 2-3 minutes.

Now, heat a suitable griddle on medium heat and add pork strips, green peppers, oil, and onion.

Cook for 5 minutes until pork is done.

Serve warm in warmed tortillas.

Nutrition:
calories 406
Protein 26 g
Carbohydrates 34 g
Fat 18 g
Cholesterol 64 mg
Sodium 376 mg
Potassium 483 mg
Phosphorus 267 mg
Calcium 57 mg
Fiber 2.4 g

Caribbean turkey curry

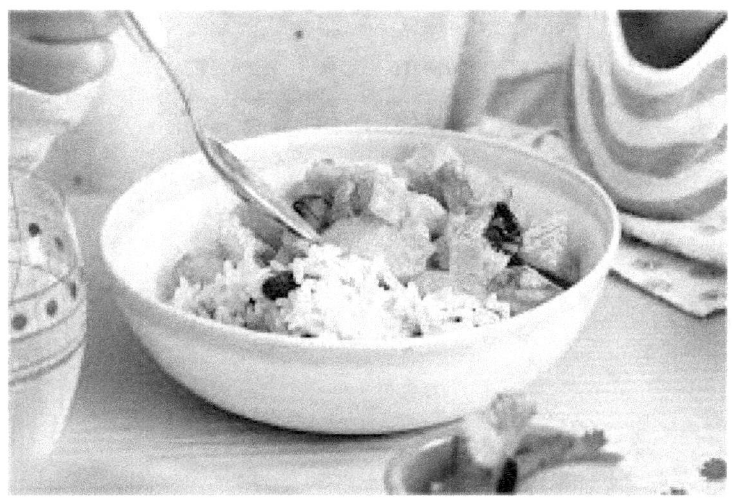

Preparation time: 10 minutes

Cooking time: 1 hour 30 minutes

Servings: 6

Ingredients:

3 1/2 lbs. turkey breast, with skin

1/4 cup butter, melted

1/4 cup honey

1 tbsp mustard

2 tsp curry powder

1 tsp garlic powder

Directions:

Place the turkey breast in a shallow roasting pan.

Insert a meat thermometer to monitor the temperature.

Bake the turkey for 1.5 hours at 350 degrees f until its internal temperature reaches 170 degrees f.

Meanwhile, thoroughly mix honey, butter, curry powder, garlic powder, and mustard in a bowl.

Glaze the cooked turkey with this mixture liberally.

Let it sit for 15 minutes for absorption.

Slice and serve.

Nutrition:
calories 275
Protein 26 g
Carbohydrates 9 g
Fat 13 g
Cholesterol 82 mg
Sodium 122 mg
Potassium 277 mg
Phosphorus 193 mg
Calcium 24 mg
Fiber 0.2 g

Chicken fajitas

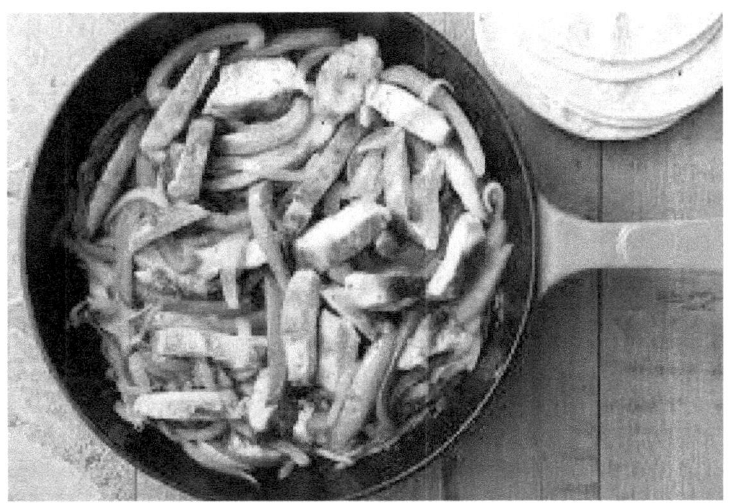

Preparation time: 10 minutes

Cooking time: 10 minutes

Servings: 8

Ingredients:

8 flour tortillas, 6" size

1/4 cup green pepper, cut in strips

1/4 cup red pepper, cut in strips

1/2 cup onion, sliced

1/2 cup cilantro

2 tbsp canola oil

12 oz boneless chicken breasts

1/4 tsp black pepper

2 tsp chili powder

1/2 tsp cumin

2 tbsp lemon juice

Directions:

Start by wrapping the tortillas in a foil.

Warm them up for 10 minutes in a preheated oven at 300 degrees f.

Add oil to a nonstick pan.

Add lemon juice chicken and seasoning

Stir fry for 5 minutes then add onion and peppers.

Continue cooking for 5 minutes or until chicken is tender.

Stir in cilantro, mix well and serve in tortillas.

Nutrition:
calories 343
Protein 24 g
Carbohydrates 33 g
Fat 13 g
Cholesterol 53 mg
Sodium 281 mg
Potassium 331 mg
Phosphorus 196 mg
Calcium 23 mg
Fiber 2.0 g

Chicken with rosemary-garlic sauce

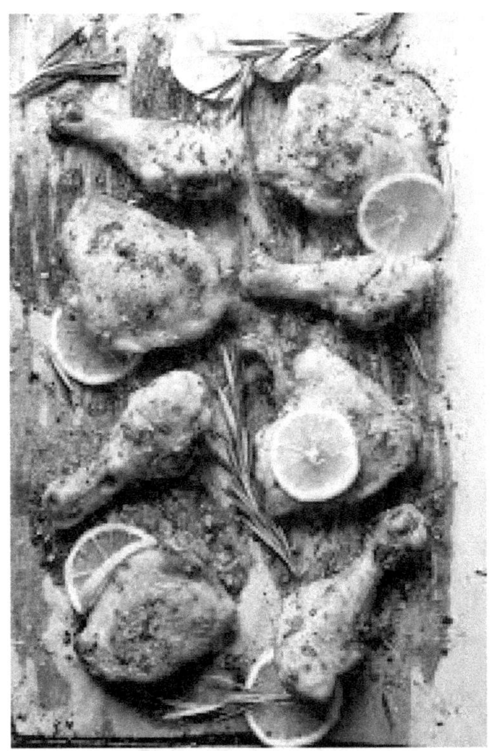

Preparation time: 10 minutes

Cooking time: 20 minutes

Servings: 8

Ingredients:

2 cups low-sodium chicken broth

1/2 cup balsamic vinegar

1/2 cup white wine

1 tbsp fresh rosemary, chopped

8 boneless, skinless chicken breasts

1 head garlic clove, chopped

2 tbsp olive or canola oil

Nonstick cooking spray

Black pepper, to taste

Directions:

Start by mixing the wine, rosemary, broth, and vinegar in a 9x13 inch baking pan.

Place the chicken breasts in it and rub the marinade into the meat. Marinate overnight.

Grease a saucepan with oil and add garlic.

Sauté until golden then set the garlic aside.

Season the marinated chicken with black pepper and sear it for 5 minutes per side until golden.

Pour the reserved marinade over it along with garlic.

Cook on reduced heat for 15 minutes and flip the chicken after 7 minutes.

Transfer the chicken to the serving plates.

Cook the remaining liquid until it thickens into a sauce.

Pour the sauce over the chicken.

Serve warm and fresh.

Nutrition:
calories 210
Protein 28 g
Carbohydrates 4 g
Fat 7 g
Cholesterol 70 mg
Sodium 85 mg
Potassium 277 mg
Phosphorus 208 mg
Calcium 26 mg
Fiber 0.2 g

Chicken paprika

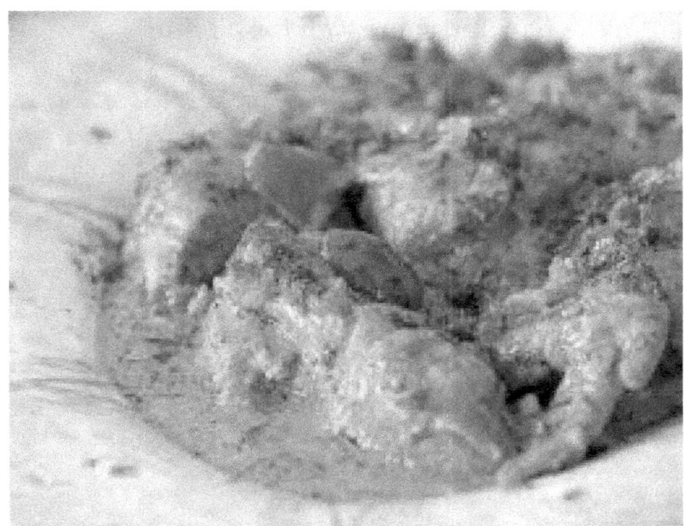

Preparation time: 10 minutes

Cooking time: 1 hour 35 minutes

Servings: 6

Ingredients:

2 tbsp canola oil

1/2 cup onion, finely chopped

1 tbsp sweet Hungarian paprika

1/2 tsp black pepper

6 chicken breasts, bone-in

2 cups of water

Cooking spray

1 cup reduced-fat sour cream

Directions:

Start by greasing a large pan with canola oil.

Add onion and sauté until golden.

Add pepper and paprika for seasoning,

Place the chicken in the pan and sauté well for 5 minutes.

Add water and then cover the pan with a suitable lid.

Let chicken simmer covered for 1.5 hours on low heat.

Stir in sour cream and mix well.

Serve warm and fresh.

Nutrition:
calories 267
Protein 30 g
Carbohydrates 3 g
Fat 15 g
Cholesterol 94 mg
Sodium 176 mg
Potassium 328 mg
Phosphorus 253 mg
Calcium 63 mg
Fiber 0.6 g

Grilled chicken marsala

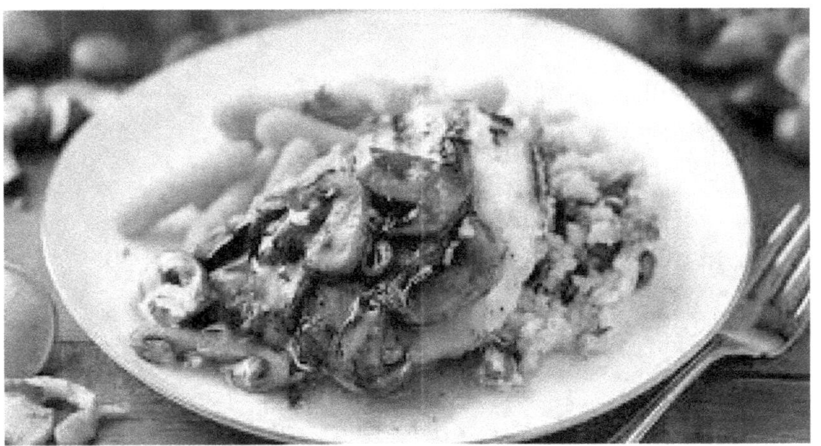

Preparation time: 10 minutes

Cooking time: 20 minutes

Servings: 4

Ingredients:

1/3 cup unsalted butter

1/2 oz sliced prosciutto, diced

2 tsp shallots, minced

2 tsp garlic, minced

1/2 cup fresh mushrooms, sliced

1/4 cup marsala wine

1-1/4 tsp ground black pepper

1 cup low-sodium chicken broth

2 tsp cornstarch

1 tsp fresh parsley, minced

2 tbsp heavy cream

1/2 tsp dried oregano

1/2 tsp dried thyme

1/2 tsp dried parsley

1/4 tsp marjoram

1/4 tsp garlic powder

1/4 tsp onion powder

4 boneless, skinless chicken breasts

2 tbsp olive oil

Directions:

Warm the butter in a saucepan over low heat.

Add prosciutto and sauté for 3 minutes.

Stir in shallots and garlic to sauté for another 30 seconds.

Now, add marsala wine and stir fry for 30 seconds.

Add mushrooms and black pepper then cook for 5 minutes on a simmer.

Mix the cornstarch with broth in a bowl and pour it into the saucepan stirring to incorporate it.

Cook for 5 minutes then add parsley and cream.

Cover the pan and let it cook for 4 minutes until it thickens.

Meanwhile, season the chicken with the remaining spices and herbs liberally.

Wrap it in a plastic wrap and pound it with a mallet. Rub the chicken with the oil.

Now, preheat a grill on medium heat and grill the chicken breast for 8 minutes per side.

Slice the grilled chicken and serve with the marsala sauce on top.

Enjoy with freshly cooked pasta.

Nutrition:
calories 581
Protein 36 g
Carbohydrates 44 g
Fat 29 g
Cholesterol 125 mg
Sodium 392 mg
Potassium 441 mg
Phosphorus 318 mg
Calcium 55 mg
Fiber 1.6 g.

Seafood recipes

Roasted salmon with gremolata

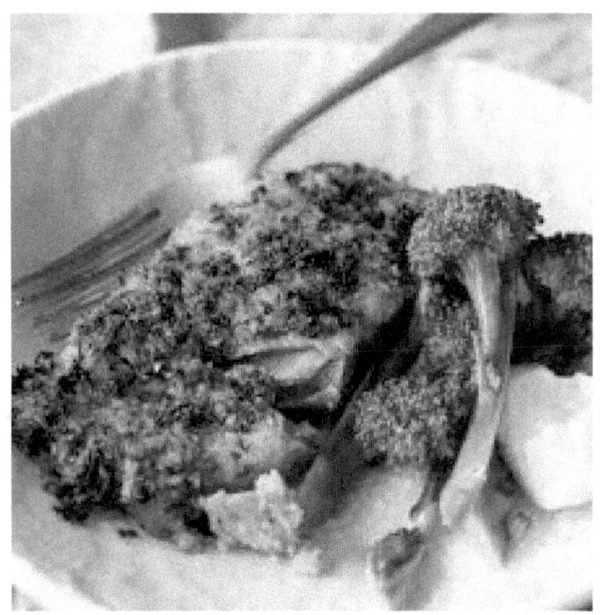

Servings: 4

Preparation Time: 15 minutes

Ingredients:

Pepper, to taste

1 lb. Salmon fillets, skinless

1 tbsp. Thyme, chopped

2 garlic cloves, minced

1 tbsp. Chopped rosemary

Zest and juice of a lemon

1/2 cup loosely packed parsley, chopped

Direction

Set your oven to 400 f.

Mix together the thyme, rosemary, garlic, lemon juice, lemon zest, and parsley in a small bowl.

Press the salmon into the herb mixture to coat them on one side. Lay the salmon on a baking pan, herb side up. Sprinkle on some pepper.

Bake them for 12 minutes. The fish should flake easily with a fork. Serve and enjoy!

Nutrition:

Calories: 170

Protein: 23 g

Sodium: 55 mg

Potassium: 626 mg

Phosphorus: 236 mg

Lime haddock

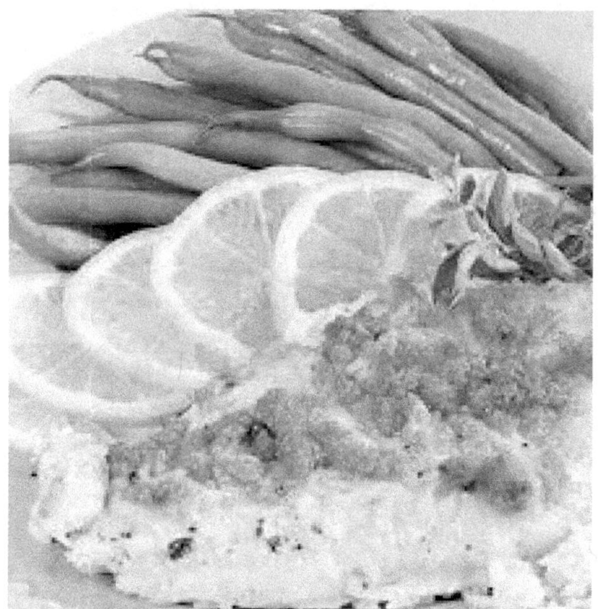

Servings: 4

Preparation Time: 15 minutes

Ingredients:

2 tsp. Chopped dill

3 tbsp. Almonds, crushed

1 tbsp. Olive oil

3 thinly sliced lime

Olive oil

Cooking spray

Pepper

Four 3 oz. Haddock fillets

Direction

Warm your oven at 400 f.

Make sure the haddock is completely dry by patting it with paper towel.

Lightly sprinkle with pepper.

Lightly spray a 9-inch casserole dish with nonstick spray.

Take the lime slices and lay them on the bottom of the baking dish. Lay the haddock on the lime.

Brush the olive oil onto the haddock and sprinkle the almonds on top.

Allow this to bake until almonds are golden and haddock is cooked through. This should take about 10 minutes.

Sprinkle the dill on top. Serve and enjoy!

Nutrition:

Calories: 124

Protein: 17 g

Sodium: 59 mg

Potassium: 283 mg

Phosphorus: 176 mg

Orange shrimp

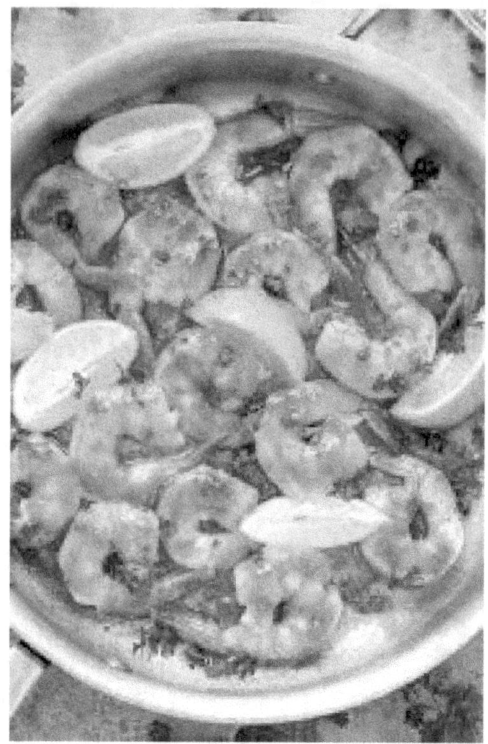

Servings: 4

Preparation Time: 10 minutes

Ingredients:

Pepper, to taste

1/2 cup orange segments

1 tsp. Unsalted butter

1 cup broccoli florets

12 oz. Deveined and peeled shrimp

1 tsp. Olive oil

1/4 tsp. Orange zest

1/2 tsp. Cornstarch

1/2 cup orange juice

Directions:

Place the orange zest, cornstarch and orange juice into a small bowl and then set aside.

Place a large pan on medium heat and heat up the oil.

Place the shrimp into the warmed skillet and cook until opaque. This will take about 5 minutes.

Place the cooked shrimp onto a plate. Place the broccoli into the skillet.

Continue cooking until broccoli is tender.

Put this on the plate with the shrimp.

Pour the orange juice into the skillet and whisk until sauce is glossy and thickened. This will take about 3 minutes.

Add in butter while whisking
Place the broccoli, shrimp, and orange segments in the skillet.

Toss everything to combine. Sprinkle with pepper. Serve and enjoy!

Nutrition:

Calories: 140

Protein: 18 g

Sodium: 130 mg

Potassium: 329 mg

Phosphorus: 196 mg

Herbed scallops

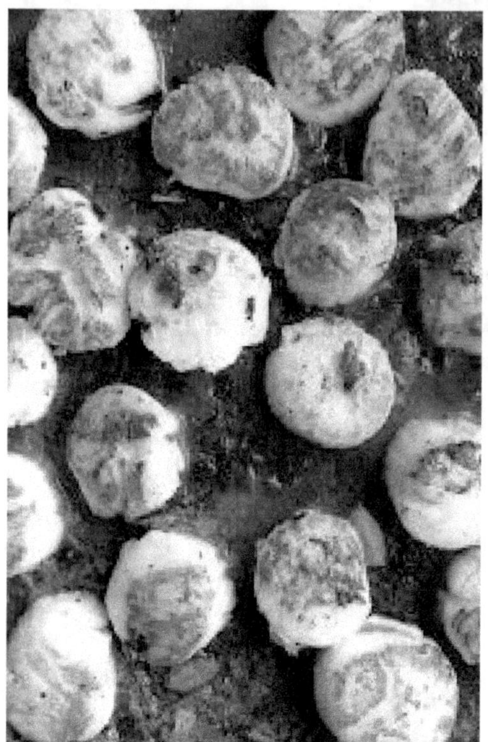

Servings: 4

Preparation Time: 10 minutes

Ingredients:

1 tsp. Chopped chives

2 tbsp. Lemon juice

Pepper, to taste

1 tsp. Chopped parsley

12 oz. Sea scallops

1 tsp. Chopped thyme

1 tbsp. Olive oil

Directions:

Place a large pan with the oil over medium heat.

Make sure the scallops are completely dry by patting them with paper towels.

Sprinkle them with pepper and place them in the warmed skillet.

Sear the scallops, turn over until browned and cooked through. This will take about 4 minutes.

Add in chives, thyme, parsley, and lemon juice. Stir to combine.

Carefully turn the scallops in the sauce to coat.

Serve immediately. Enjoy!

Nutrition:

Calories: 131

Protein: 14 g

Sodium: 136 mg

Potassium: 268 mg

Phosphorus: 176 mg

Almond sole

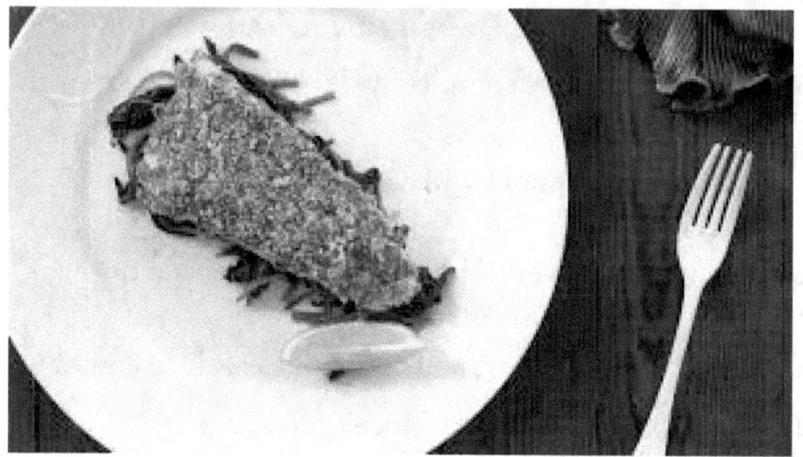

Servings: 4

Preparation Time: 10 minutes

Ingredients:

1 tsp. Olive oil

1 tbsp. Chopped parsley

3 tbsp. Almond flour

Pepper, to taste

1 tsp. Thyme, chopped

Four 3 oz. Sole fillets

Directions:

Preheat oven to 350 f. Line a baking sheet with parchment paper.

Make sure the sole is completely dry by patting them with paper towels.

Sprinkle the sole fillets with pepper.

Place thyme, parsley, and almond flour into a shallow bowl and mix until blended.

Brush the sole with olive oil. Dredge with the almond flour.

Put the sole onto the baking sheet.

Allow this to bake for 15 minutes or until the sole is opaque.

Serve immediately. Enjoy!

Nutrition:

Calories: 113

Protein: 17 g

Sodium: 70 mg

Potassium: 327 mg

Phosphorus: 168 mg

Garlic butter tilapia

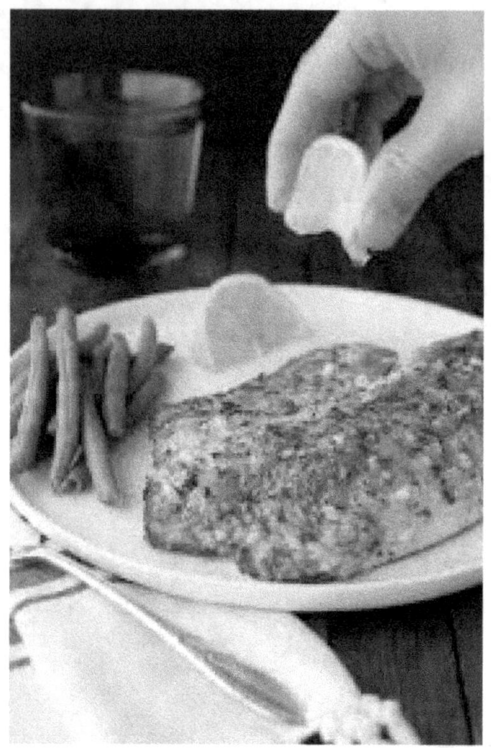

Servings: 4

Preparation Time: 15 minutes

Ingredients:

Pepper, to taste

Four 3 oz. Tilapia fillets

1 tbsp. Olive oil

1 tbsp. Plain flour

Zest and juice of 1/2 lemon

1 tsp. Minced garlic

2 tbsp. Chopped parsley

1 minced shallot

1/4 cup melted unsalted butter

Directions:

Preheat your oven to 400 f. Make sure the tilapia is completely dry by patting it with paper towels.

Put flour, parsley, lemon zest, garlic, lemon juice, shallot and butter in a small bowl and mix well. Set aside.

Add oil in an oven-safe large skillet over medium heat.

Sprinkle the pepper on the fillets. Place the tilapia into the skillet and brown the tilapia. Turn it once. This should take no more than 4 minutes.

Pour the butter mixture over the tilapia and put the skillet into the oven.

Bake until just turning opaque in the middle. This will take around 4 minutes.

Remove from oven and place on plates.

Serve with some sauce from the skillet. Enjoy!

Nutrition:

Calories: 219

Protein: 17 g

Sodium: 45 mg

Potassium: 252 mg

Phosphorus: 149 mg

Salmon in foil

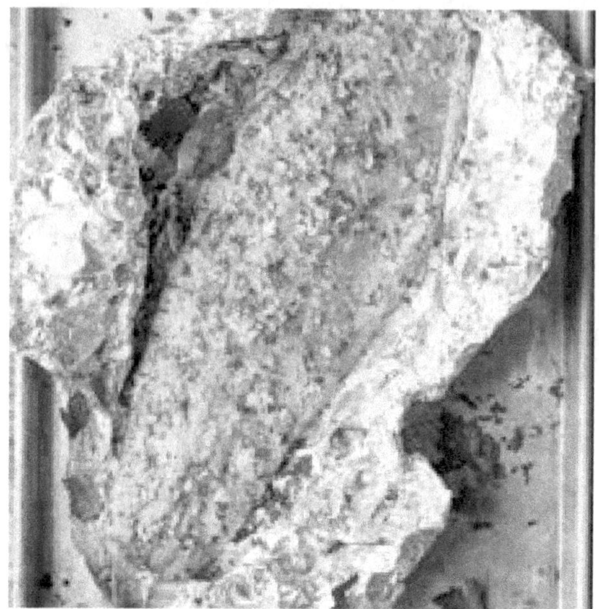

Servings: 4

Preparation Time: 30 minutes

Ingredients:

2 tsp. Peeled and grated ginger

Juice from 1 lemon

Four 2 oz. Salmon fillet

1 chopped scallion

8 asparagus spears

1 sliced bell pepper

2 cups bean sprouts

Directions:

Preheat oven to 400 f.

Cut 4 pieces of foil that are about one-foot square.

Cut the asparagus into 2-inch pieces.

Divide out the scallion, asparagus, bell pepper, and bean sprouts evenly across the foil pieces.

Put one salmon fillet on top of each vegetable pile.

Add ginger and lemon juice into a small bowl and stir to combine. Cover the salmon with this mixture.

Fold the foil over the salmon and seal each packet and put them on the baking sheet.

Allow this to bake until fish flakes easily. This will take about 20 minutes.

Serve immediately. Enjoy!

Oven-fried fish with pineapple salsa

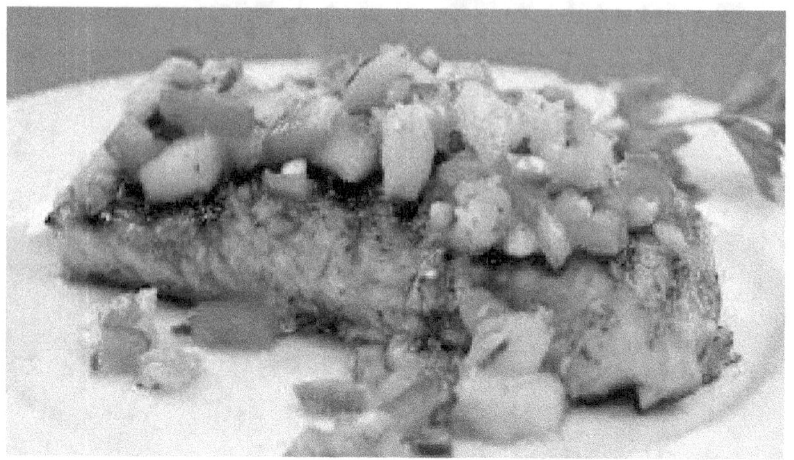

Servings: 4

Preparation Time: 30 minutes

Ingredients:

For the salsa:

1/4 cup chopped cilantro

Lime juice from 1/2 lime

1/2 jalapeno pepper, seeded and diced

1/4 cup red onion, diced

1 cup pineapple, diced

For the fish:

1 tbsp. Butter

2 tbsp. Unsweetened rice milk

1 egg, beaten

1/4 cup all-purpose flour

1/4 cup yellow cornmeal

1/2 tsp. Paprika

1/2 tsp. Garlic powder

1 lb. Whitefish fillets

Directions

Mix all of the salsa ingredients together in a bowl. Place to the side while you fix the fish.

Preheat oven to 400 f and grease a baking dish with the butter.

Rub the fish fillets with paprika and garlic powder.

Combine the flour and cornmeal.

In a separate bowl, mix the egg and milk together.

Dip the fish into the egg mixture and then coat them with the flour mixture. Lay the fish in the prepared dish.

Bake the fish for 20 minutes. Flip them once, halfway through the cooking process. The fish should be golden and flake easily with a fork.

Serve the fish with the pineapple salsa on top. Enjoy!

Nutrition:

Calories: 242

Protein: 27 g

Sodium: 83 mg

Potassium: 474 mg

Phosphorus: 238 mg

Lemon garlic halibut

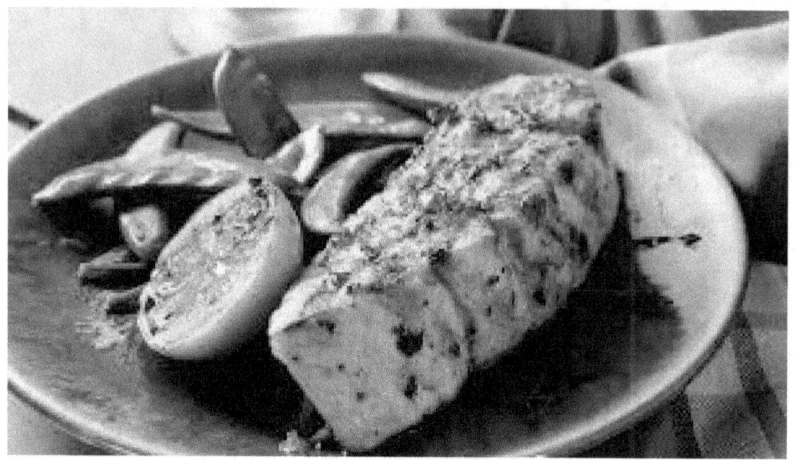

Servings: 4

Preparation Time: 30 minutes

Ingredients:

2 tbsp. Chopped parsley

Zest of a lemon

1 lb. Halibut fillets, skin removed

Pepper, to taste

2 tbsp. Cilantro, chopped

2 garlic cloves, minced

2 tbsp. Evo, divided

1/4 cup lemon juice

Directions:

Set your oven to 400 f.

Mix together the garlic, lemon juice, a tbsp. Olive oil and some pepper.

Add the halibut to the bowl and flip it around to make sure that it is coated well. Let this marinate for 10 minutes.

Lay the fillets on a baking pan and brush some more of the marinade over the top. Let the fish bake for 12 to 15 minutes.

You can brush the fish with the marinade halfway through the cooking process. The fish is done when it can be flaked easily with a fork.

Discard any of the leftover marinade.

Serve the fish with some parsley, cilantro, and lemon zest. Enjoy!

Nutrition:

Calories: 169

Protein: 21 g

Sodium: 79 mg

Potassium: 528 mg

Phosphorus: 272 mg

Shrimp fried rice

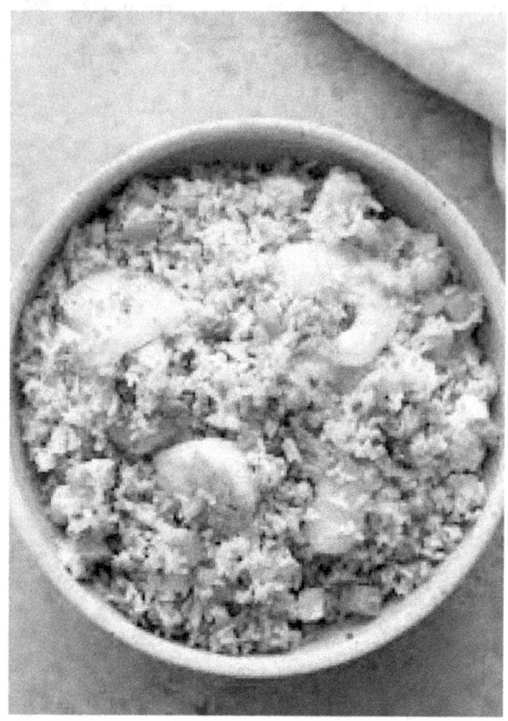

Servings: 6

Preparation Time: 15 minutes

Ingredients:

3 cups cooked rice

1 cup sugar snap peas

1 lb. Deveined and peeled shrimp

3 garlic cloves, minced

2-inch piece minced ginger

1/2 chopped sweet onion

1 tbsp. Evo

Directions:

Over medium heat, add oil in a wok or a large pan.

Place in the onion and stir constantly for around 3 to 5 minutes. The onion should soften.

Add in the garlic and ginger, and stir the mixture until it becomes fragrant.

Add in the shrimp and cook until the shrimp has turned opaque and is almost cooked through about 5 minutes.

Mix in the rice and snap peas, stirring until everything is well mixed and heated through. Serve and enjoy!

Nutrition:

Calories: 217

Protein: 13 g

Sodium: 431 mg

Potassium: 157 mg

Phosphorus: 226 mg

Shrimp and Bok choy

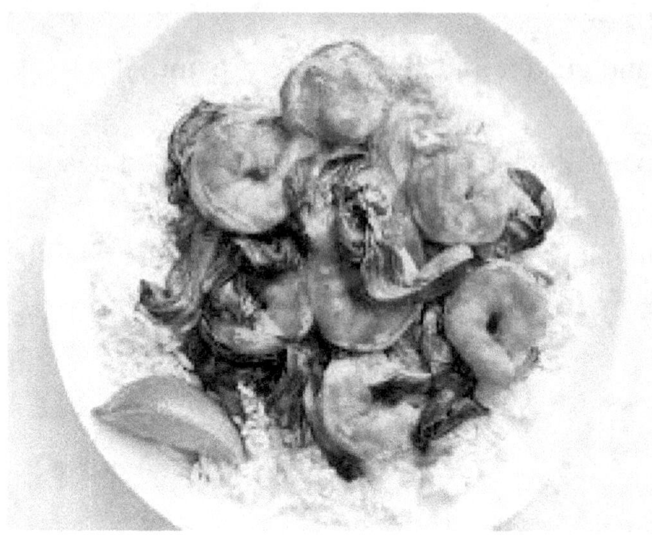

Servings: 6

Preparation Time: 25 minutes

Ingredients:

2 thinly sliced scallions

2 tbsp. Lime juice

1 lb. Thinly sliced Bok choy

2 tbsp. Rice vinegar

2 tsp. Honey

2-inch piece minced ginger

3 minced ginger cloves

1 tsp. Toasted sesame oil

12 oz. Deveined and peeled shrimp

1/4 cup cilantro, chopped

Thinly sliced jalapeno pepper

Directions:

Set your oven to 375 f.

Mix together the ginger, garlic and shrimp in a small bowl.

In a separate bowl, mix together the rice vinegar, honey, lime juice and sesame oil.

Cut out 4 large circles from parchment paper. It should be at least 12 inches in diameter.

On each circle, place a handful of Bok choy and top with the shrimp and the garlic mixture, jalapeno slices, and scallions.

Drizzle each with a quarter of the lime mixture.

Fold up the parchment paper and roll the edges together to create a seal.

Lay the packets on a baking pan and bake for 15 minutes.

Take it out of the oven and allow it to rest for 5 minutes. Be careful when opening the packet so that you don't get burned by steam. Garnish with cilantro and serve with rice. Enjoy!

Nutrition:

Calories: 92

Protein: 12 g

Sodium: 484 mg

Potassium: 162 mg

Phosphorus: 217 mg

Shrimp skewers with mango salsa

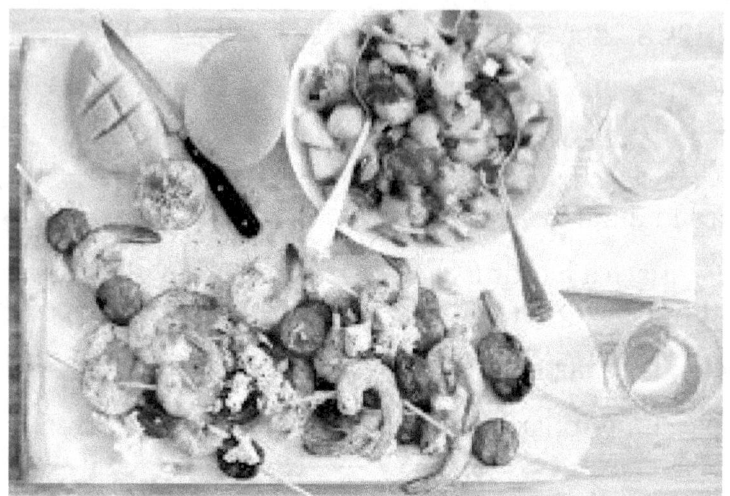

Servings: 6

Preparation Time: 50 minutes

Ingredients:

For the shrimp:

1 tsp. Canola oil

1 lb. Cleaned shrimp, tails on

1-inch piece ginger, minced

2 tbsp. Honey

Lime juice of 2 limes

For the salsa:

Small red chili, diced

1/4 cup sweet onion, diced

Juice of a lime

Diced and peeled mango

Diced and seeded medium size cucumber

Directions:

For the shrimp: mix together the ginger, honey and lime juice. Toss the shrimp to coat with the mixture.

Cover the shrimp and refrigerate them for a minimum of 30 minutes.

Thread the shrimp onto your skewers.

Heat up your grill to medium high and brush with some oil.

Cook your skewers for 3 to 6 minutes on both sides. The shrimp should turn opaque when cooked through.

For the salsa: toss the lime juice, mango, cucumber, chili, and onion together in a small bowl.

Once the shrimp is cooked, remove from skewers and add to salsa. Toss together and serve. Enjoy!

Nutrition:

Calories: 123

Protein: 11 g

Sodium: 431 mg

Potassium: 317 mg

Phosphorus: 213 mg

Salads & sauces

Pear & brie salad

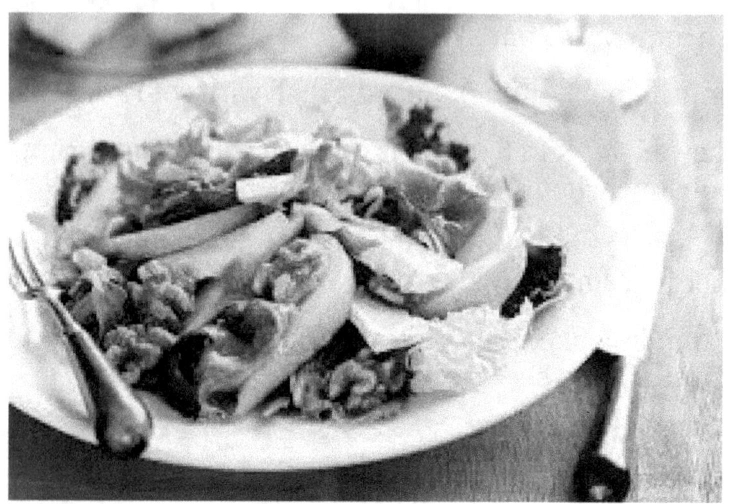

Servings: 4
preparation time: 5 minutes
cooking time: 4 minutes

1/4 cucumber

/2 cup canned pears, juices drained

1 cup arugula

1/4 cup brie, chopped

1/2 lemon

1 tbsp olive oil

Peel and dice the cucumber.

Dice the pear.

Wash the arugula.

Combine salad in a serving bowl and crumble the brie over the top.

Whisk the olive oil and lemon juice together.

Drizzle over the salad.

Season with a little black pepper to taste and serve immediately.

Nutrition:
Calories 54

Protein 1 g

Carbohydrates 12 g

Fat 7 g

Sodium 57mg

Potassium 115 mg

Phosphorus 67 mg

Kidney-friendly chips

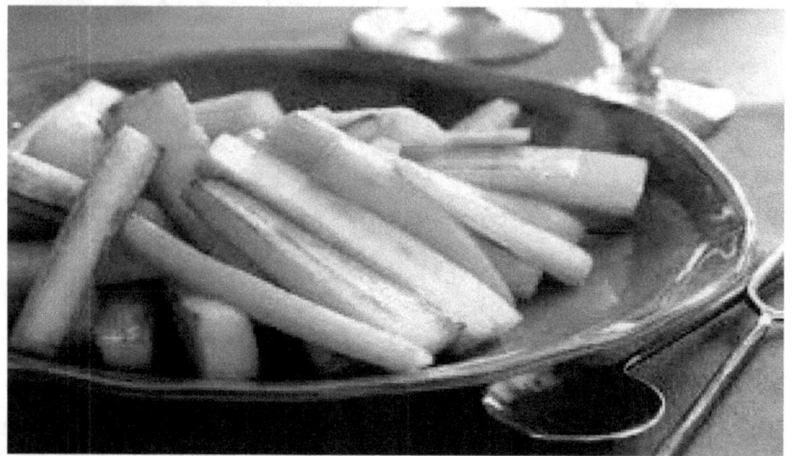

Servings: 4
preparation time: 5 minutes
cooking time: 50 minutes

4 parsnips, peeled and sliced

1 tbsp extra virgin olive oil

1 tsp black pepper

1 tsp thyme

1 tsp chili flakes

Heat oven to 375°f/190°c/gas mark 5.

Grease a baking tray with the olive oil.

Add the parsnip slices in a thin layer.

Sprinkle over the thyme and chili slices and toss to coat.

Bake for 40-50 minutes (turning half way through to ensure even crispiness!)

Nutrition:
Calories 62

Protein 0g

Carbohydrates 5 g

Fat 3 g

Sodium 7 mg

Potassium 115 mg

Phosphorus 112 mg

Spaghetti squash puree

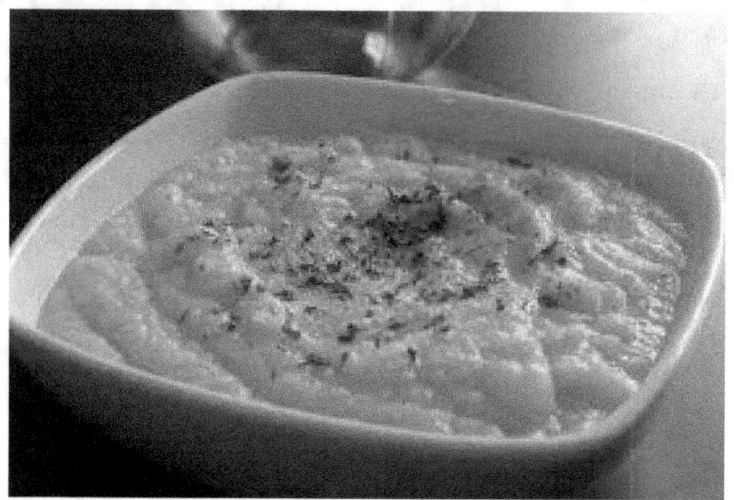

Servings: 8
preparation time: 10 minutes
cooking time: 45 minutes

1 spaghetti squash (approx. 4 cups)

1 tsp chili flakes

3 tbsp parsley, finely chopped

1 tbsp extra virgin olive oil

Pre-heat the oven to 375°f/190 °c/gas mark 5.

Cut squash in half lengthways.

Place each side into a large oven dish (skin up).

Pour half a cup of water into the dish.

Bake for 45 minutes or until tender.

Remove from the oven and allow to cool.

Flake with a fork to shred the flesh into a bowl.

Stir in the chili flakes, black pepper, parsley and garlic cloves.

Blend in a food processor until smooth.

Serve on your favorite salad or with your favorite meat.

Nutrition:
Calories 32

Protein 0 g

Carbohydrates 4 g

Fat 2 g

Sodium 16 mg

Potassium 71 mg

Phosphorus 13 mg

Mexican rice

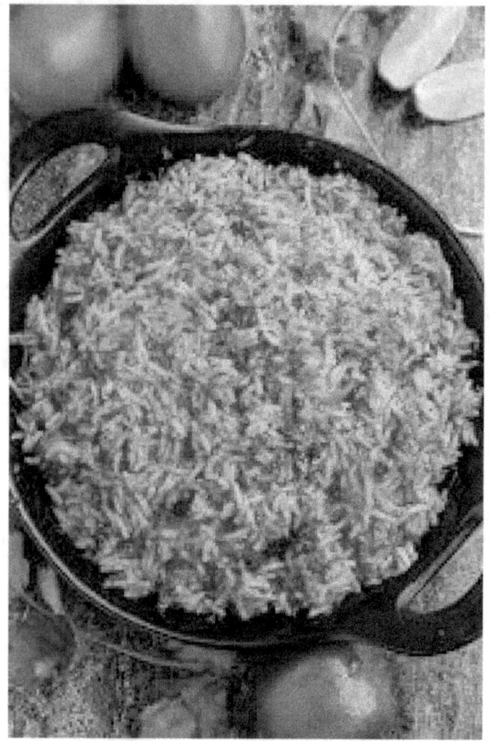

Servings: 4
preparation time: 5 minutes
cooking time: 25 minutes

1 cup low-sodium chicken broth

1 cup water

1 cup uncooked rice

1 tbsp extra virgin olive oil

1 red onion, chopped

1 tbsp cilantro, chopped

1 red pepper, finely diced

1 lemon

Add the stock, water and rice into a saucepan and boil over a high heat.

Reduce the heat and simmer for 25 minutes until rice is cooked and the liquid is nearly absorbed.

Meanwhile, heat the oil in a skillet on a medium heat and sauté the onion until soft.

Add the peppers and cook for another 10 minutes.

Stir the onions and peppers into the rice and beans and then squeeze in the lemon juice and top with cilantro to serve.

Nutrition:
Calories

Protein 4 g

Carbohydrates 12 g

Fat 3 g

Sodium 9 mg

Potassium 9 mg

Phosphorus 47 mg

Lemony green beans

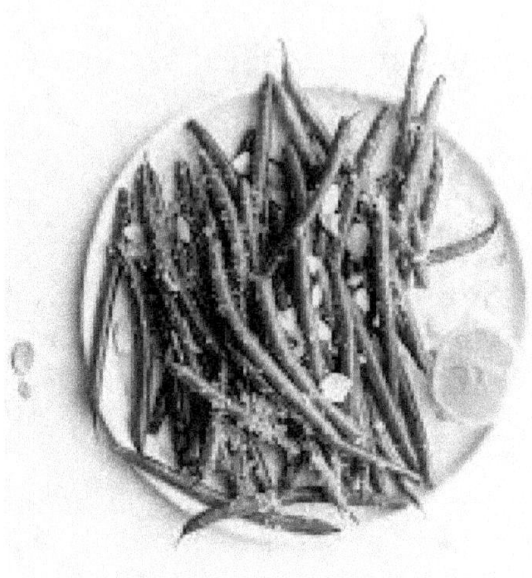

Servings: 4
preparation time: 5 minutes
cooking time: 20 minutes

1 cup green beans

1 tbsp unsalted butter

1 lemon

Pinch black pepper

Steam the green beans over a high heat for 15-20 minutes or until soft.

Drain and place to one side to cool.

Heat the butter in a small pan until melted.

Whisk in the lemon juice.

Pour over the broccoli stems, cover and allow to set the fridge for 30 minutes.

Serve with a pinch of black pepper.

Nutrition:
Calories 34

Protein 0 g

Carbohydrates 2 g

Fat 2 g

Sodium 2 mg

Potassium 60 mg

Phosphorus 10 mg

Arugula pesto

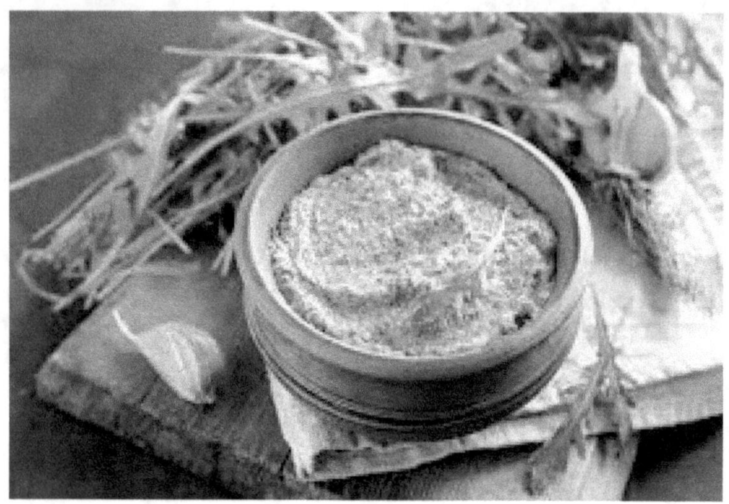

Servings: 5
preparation time: 5 minutes
cooking time: Na

5 tbsp fresh basil

1 cup arugula

1 cup baby spinach

1 tsp black pepper

1/4 cup extra virgin olive oil

2 garlic cloves

1 lemon, juiced

1/4 cup brie (optional)

Blend all ingredients in a food processor or a blender to reach required texture - chunky for a rustic feel or smooth as a dressing

Store in an airtight container in the fridge for 3-4 days.

Can be added to pasta for a delicious sauce, used as a dip with your favorite bread and served over a salad.

Nutrition:
Calories 132

Protein 1 g

Carbohydrates 0 g

Fat 13 g

Sodium 50 mg

Potassium 36 mg

Phosphorus 51 mg

Brie & beetroot salad

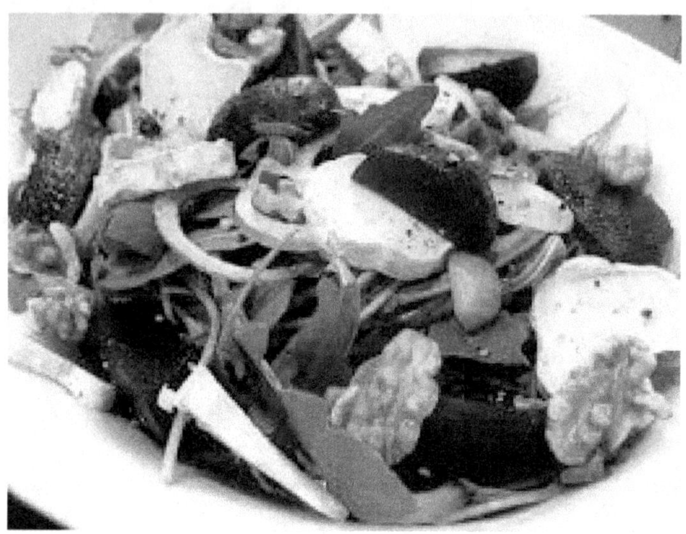

Servings: 2
preparation time: 5 minutes
cooking time: n/a

1/2 cup brie

1 cup baby spinach leaves, washed

1/2 cup canned beets, juices drained & sliced

Pinch black pepper

1 tbsp olive oil

1/4 cucumber, peeled and diced

Chop the brie into bite-size pieces.

Add all of the ingredients to a salad bowl and toss.

Serve right away.

Hint: if preparing the salad in advance, wait until just before
serving to dress with olive oil or the salad will wilt.

Nutrition:
Calories 283

Protein 14 g

Carbohydrates 3 g

Fat 23 g

Sodium 483 mg

Potassium 394 mg

Phosphorus 241 mg

Eggplant dip

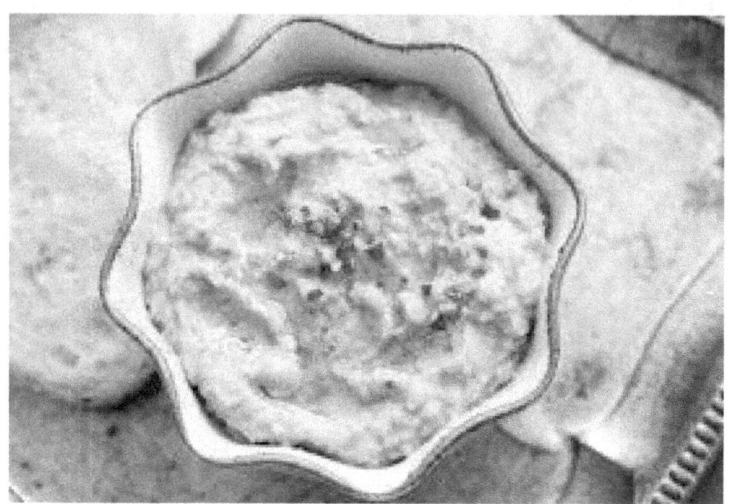

Servings: 4
preparation time: 5 minutes
cooking time: 30 minutes

2 eggplants (approx. 4 cups)

2 tbsp extra virgin olive oil

2 garlic cloves, minced

1/2 onion. Finely diced

1 tsp cumin

1 tsp turmeric

1 tbsp parsley

Pinch black pepper

Preheat the broiler/grill to a medium heat.

Slice the eggplants in half and add to a baking tray.

Drizzle over 1 tbsp olive oil and sprinkle over a pinch a black pepper.

Place under the grill for 15-20 minutes or until eggplants are soft and lightly grilled.

Now heat 1 tbsp oil in a skillet over a medium-high heat.

Add onions and garlic and sauté for 5 minutes or until soft.

Now add the cumin, followed by the turmeric and stir to release the aromas.

Turn the heat right down.

Now remove the eggplant and allow to cool slightly before scooping out the flesh.

Roughly chop with a sharp knife and add to the pan with the onions and garlic.

Sauté for 10 minutes and remove from the heat.

Allow to cool before blending in a food processor and adding parsley.

Enjoy as a healthy dip.

Nutrition:
Calories 70

Protein 2 g

Carbohydrates 9 g

Fat 3 g

Sodium 4 mg

Potassium 269 mg

Phosphorus 20 mg

Char-grilled veg salad

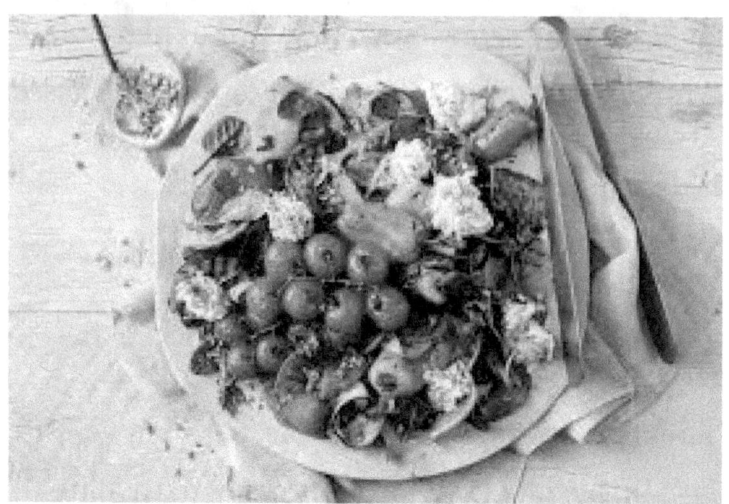

Servings: 4
preparation time: 5 minutes
cooking time: 20 minutes

Another delicious side dishes.

1 eggplant, sliced (approx. 2 cups

2 tbsp olive oil

1 zucchini, peeled & sliced

2 diced red bell peppers, sliced

1/2 cup spinach leaves

Pinch of pepper

Pre-heat a griddle pan over a high heat and add the eggplant slices for 10 minutes, turning over half way through, until lightly charred.

Remove from the pan and place to one side.

Now add a little olive oil and the zucchini and pepper slices.

Repeat above.

Mix all of the ingredients together.

Toss together and serve.

Nutrition:
Calories 79

Protein 0 g

Carbohydrates 3 g

Fat 6 g

Sodium 4 mg

Potassium 215 mg

Phosphorus 54 mg

Crab & scallion salad

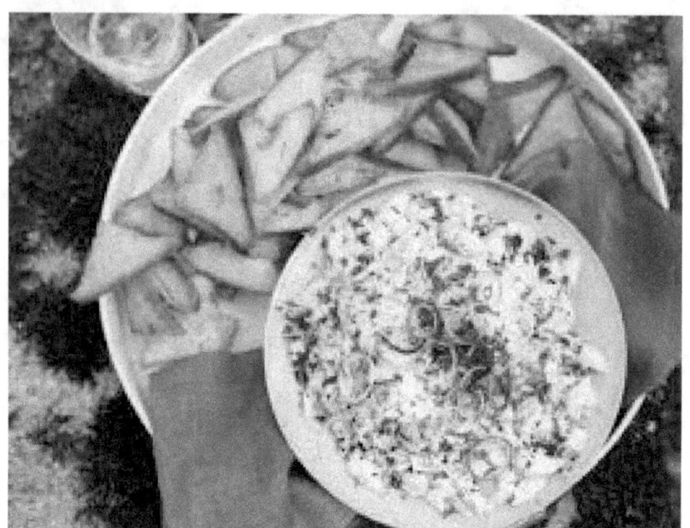

Servings: 4
preparation time: 5 minutes
cooking time: Na

A chunky salad on the side.

8oz crab meat

Juice of 1 lemon

Pinch of pepper

1 cup arugula, washed

1/4 cup scallions, washed and sliced

1 tbsp of olive oil

Mix the crab meat and lemon juice together.

Season with pepper and place to one side.

Into a salad bowl, add the arugula and scallions.

Drizzle with the olive oil and toss to coat.

Mix the crab meat with the salad and serve.

Nutrition:
Calories 81

Protein 9 g

Carbohydrates 0 g

Fat 4 g

Sodium 286 mg

Potassium 197 mg

Phosphorus 86 mg

Beautiful beetroot sauce

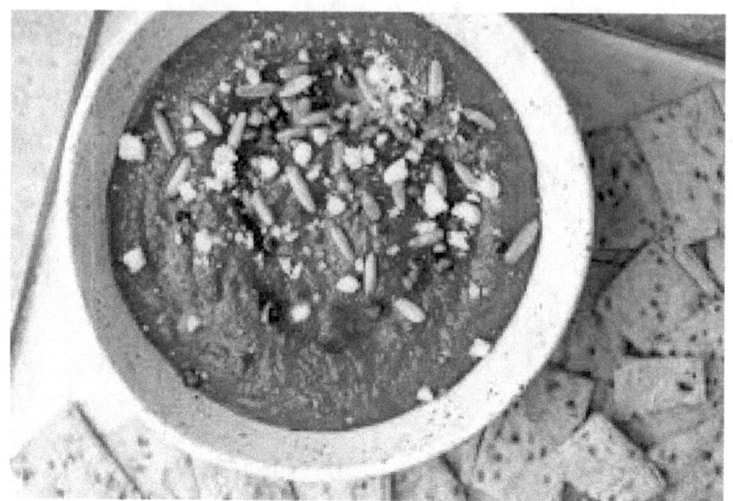

Servings: 4
preparation time: 5 minutes
cooking time: 15 minutes

Great as a dip, with curries or even as a salad topper.

1 cup of canned beetroot, no added sugar or salt

1 juiced lemon

1 tsp dry mustard

A pinch of black pepper to taste

Add all of the ingredients to a blender and puree until smooth.

Serve immediately or store in an airtight container in the fridge for 2-3 days.

Nutrition:
Calories 25

Protein 0 g

Carbohydrates 4 g

Fat 0 g

Sodium 35 mg

Potassium 15 mg

Phosphorus 15 mg

Vegetarian dishes

Egg white frittata with penne

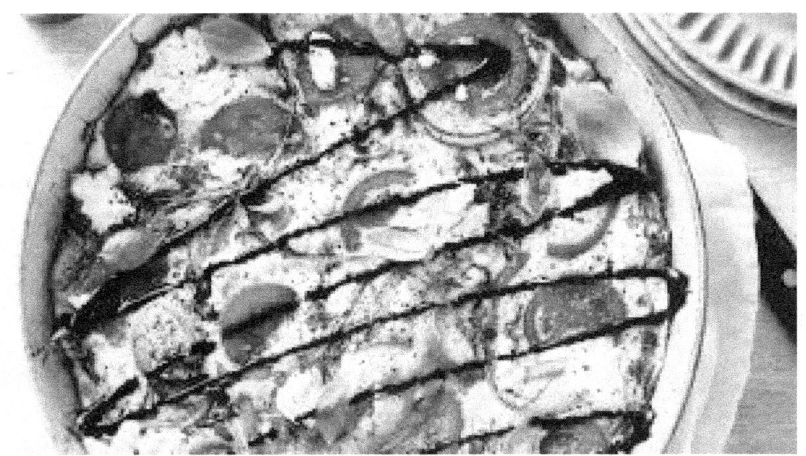

Preparation time: 15 minutes

Cooking time: 30 minutes

Serving: 4

Ingredients

Egg whites- 6

Rice milk – ¼ cup

Chopped fresh parsley – 1 tbsp

Chopped fresh thyme – 1 tsp

Chopped fresh chives – 1 tsp

Ground black pepper

Olive oil – 2 tsp.

Small sweet onion – ¼, chopped

Minced garlic – 1 tsp

Boiled and chopped red bell pepper – ½ cup

Cooked penne – 2 cups

Directions:

Preheat the oven to 350f.

In a bowl, whisk together the egg whites, rice milk, parsley, thyme, chives, and pepper.

Heat the oil in a skillet.

Sauté the onion, garlic, red pepper for 4 minutes or until they are softened.

Add the cooked penne to the skillet.

Pour the egg mixture over the pasta and shake the pan to coat the pasta.

Leave the skillet on the heat for 1 minute to set the bottom of the frittata and then transfer the skillet to the oven.

Bake the frittata for 25 minutes, or until it is set and golden brown.

Serve.

Nutrition:

Calories: 170

Fat: 3g

Carb: 25g

Phosphorus: 62mg

Potassium: 144mg

Sodium: 90mg

Protein: 10g

Vegetable fried rice

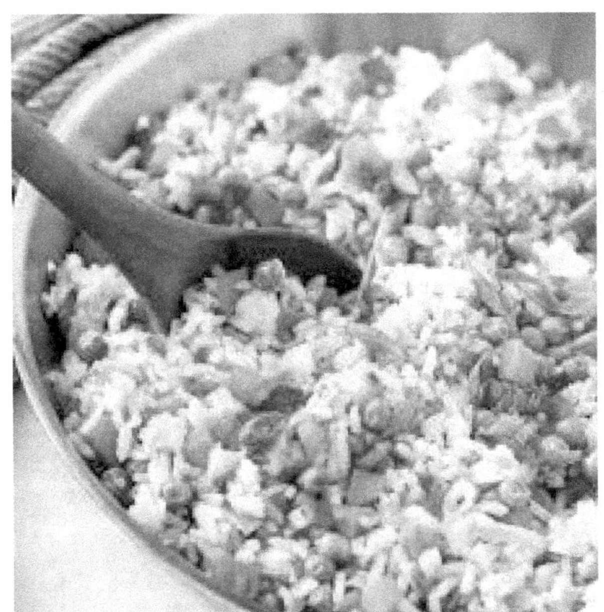

Preparation time: 20 minutes

Cooking time: 20 minutes

Serving: 6

Ingredients

Olive oil – 1 tbsp

Sweet onion – ½, chopped

Grated fresh ginger – 1 tbsp

Minced garlic - 2 tsp

Sliced carrots – 1 cup

Chopped eggplant – ½ cup

Peas – ½ cup

Green beans – ½ cup, cut into 1-inch pieces

Chopped fresh cilantro – 2 tbsp

Cooked rice – 3 cups

Directions:

Heat the olive oil in a skillet.

Sauté the ginger, onion, and garlic for 3 minutes or until softened.

Stir in carrot, eggplant, green beans, and peas and sauté for 3 minutes more.

Add cilantro and rice.

Sauté, constantly stirring, for about 10 minutes or until the rice is heated through.

Serve.

Nutrition:

Calories: 189

Fat: 7g

Carb: 28g

Phosphorus: 89mg

Potassium: 172mg

Sodium: 13mg

Protein: 6g

Bulgur-stuffed spaghetti squash

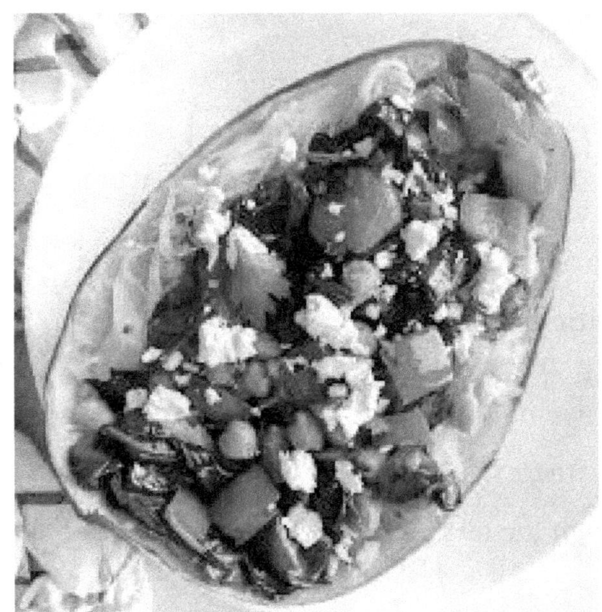

Preparation time: 30 minutes

Cooking time: 50 minutes

Serving: 4

Ingredients for the squash

Spaghetti squash – 2 smalls halved

Olive oil – 1 tsp

Ground black pepper

For the filling

Olive oil – 1 tsp

Small sweet onion – ½, finely chopped

Minced garlic – 1 tsp

Chopped carrot – ½ cup

Cranberries – ½ cup

Chopped fresh thyme – 1 tsp

Ground cumin – ½ tsp.

Ground coriander – ½ tsp

Juice of ½ lemon

Cooked bulgur – 1 cup

Directions:

To make the squash, preheat the oven to 350f.

Line a baking sheet with parchment paper.

Lightly oil the cut sides of the squash, season with pepper, and place them cut side down on the baking sheet.

Bake for 25 to 30 minutes, or until tender.

Remove the squash from the oven and flip the squash halves over.

Scoop out the flesh from each half, leaving about ½ inch around the edges and keeping the skin intact.

Place 2 cups of squash flesh in a bowl and reserve the rest for another recipe.

To make the filling: in a skillet, heat the olive oil.

Sauté the onion, carrot, garlic, and cranberries for 5 to 6 minutes or until softened.

Add the sautéed vegetables to the squash in the bowl.

Add the thyme, cumin, and coriander, stirring to combine.

Stir in the lemon juice and cooked bulgur until well mixed.

Spoon the filling evenly into the squash halves.

Bake in the oven for 15 minutes, or until heated through.

Serve.

Nutrition:

Calories: 111

Fat: 2g

Carb: 17g

Phosphorus: 38mg

Potassium: 182mg

Sodium: 22mg

Protein: 3g

Couscous burgers

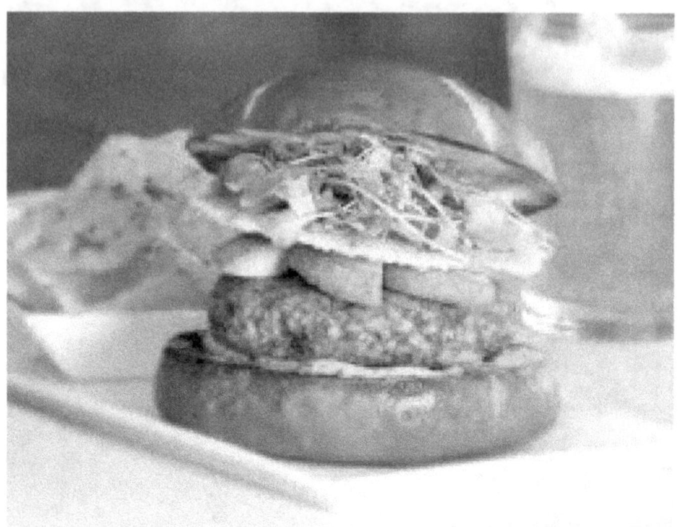

Preparation time: 20 minutes

Cooking time: 10 minutes

Serving: 4

Ingredients

Canned chickpeas – ½ cup, rinsed and drained

Chopped fresh cilantro – 2 tbsp

Chopped fresh parsley

Lemon juice - 1 tbsp

Lemon zest – 2 tsp

Minced garlic – 1 tsp

Cooked couscous – 2 ½ cups

Eggs – 2, lightly beaten

Olive oil – 2 tbsp.

Directions:

Put the cilantro, chickpeas, parsley, lemon juice, lemon zest, and garlic in a food processor and pulse until a paste form.

Transfer the chickpea mixture to a bowl, and add the eggs and couscous. Mix well.

Chill the mixture in the refrigerator for 1 hour.

Form the couscous mixture into 4 patties.

Heat olive oil in a skillet.

Place the patties in the skillet, 2 at a time, gently pressing them down with the fork of a spatula.

Cook for 5 minutes or until golden, and flip the patties over.

Cook the other side for 5 minutes and transfer the cooked burgers to a plate covered with a paper towel.

Repeat with the remaining 2 burgers.

Nutrition:

Calories: 242

Fat: 10g

Carb: 29g

Phosphorus: 108mg

Potassium: 168mg

Sodium: 43mg

Protein: 9g

Marinated tofu stir-fry

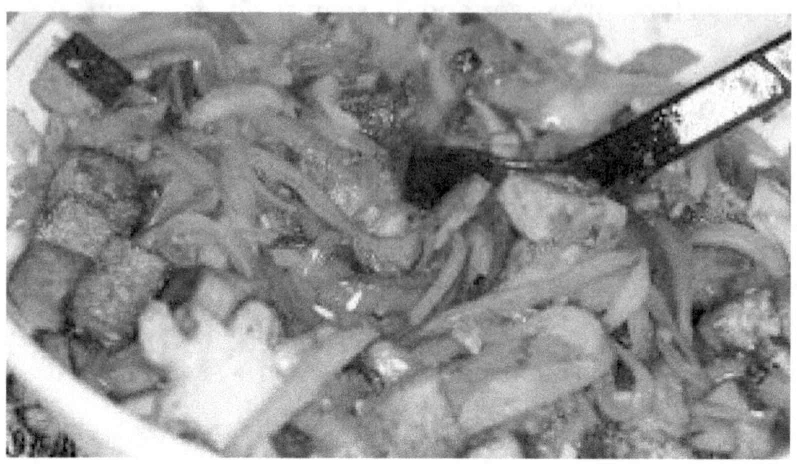

Preparation time: 20 minutes

Cooking time: 20 minutes

Serving: 4

Ingredients for the tofu

Lemon juice – 1 tbsp

Minced garlic – 1 tsp

Grated fresh ginger – 1 tsp

Pinch red pepper flakes

Extra-firm tofu- 5 ounces, pressed well and cubed

For the stir-fry

Olive oil – 1 tbsp

Cauliflower florets – ½ cup

Thinly sliced carrots – ½ cup

Julienned red pepper – ½ cup

Fresh green beans – ½ cup

Cooked white rice – 2 cups

Directions:

In a bowl, mix the lemon juice, garlic, ginger, and red pepper flakes.

Add the tofu and toss to coat.

Place the bowl in the refrigerator and marinate for 2 hours.

To make the stir-fry, heat the oil in a skillet.

Sauté the tofu for 8 minutes or until it is lightly browned and heated through.

Add the carrots, and cauliflower and sauté for 5 minutes. Stirring and tossing constantly.

Add the red pepper and green beans, sauté for 3 minutes more.

Serve over white rice.

Nutrition:

Calories: 190

Fat: 6g

Carb: 30g

Phosphorus: 90mg

Potassium: 199mg

Sodium: 22mg

Protein: 6g

Thai-inspired vegetable curry

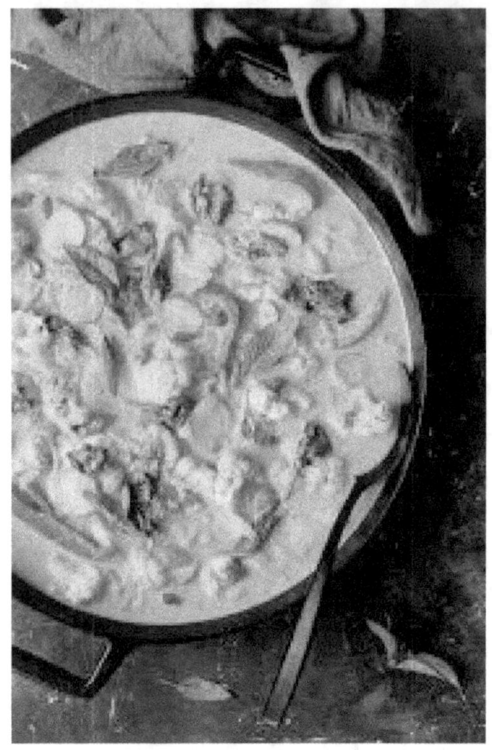

Preparation time: 15 minutes

Cooking time: 45 minutes

Serving: 4

Ingredients

Olive oil – 2 tsp

Sweet onion – ½, diced

Minced garlic – 2 tsp

Grated fresh ginger – 2 tsp

Eggplant – ½, peeled and diced

Carrot – 1, peeled and diced

Red bell pepper – 1, diced

Hot curry powder – 1 tbsp.

Ground cumin – 1 tsp

Coriander – ½ tsp

Pinch cayenne pepper

Homemade vegetable stock – 1 ½ cups

Cornstarch – 1 tbsp

Water – ¼ cup

Directions:

Heat the oil in a stockpot.

Sauté the ginger, garlic, and onion for 3 minutes or until they are softened.

Add the red pepper, carrots, eggplant, and stir often for 6 minutes.

Stir in the cumin, curry powder, coriander, cayenne pepper, and vegetable stock.

Bring the curry to a boil and then lower the heat to low.

Simmer the curry for 30 minutes or until the vegetables are tender.

In a bowl, stir together the cornstarch and water.

Stir in the cornstarch mixture into the curry and simmer for 5 minutes or until the sauce has thickened.

Nutrition:

Calories: 100

Fat: 3g

Carb: 9g

Phosphorus: 28mg

Potassium: 180mg

Sodium: 218mg

Protein: 1g

Linguine with roasted red pepper-basil sauce

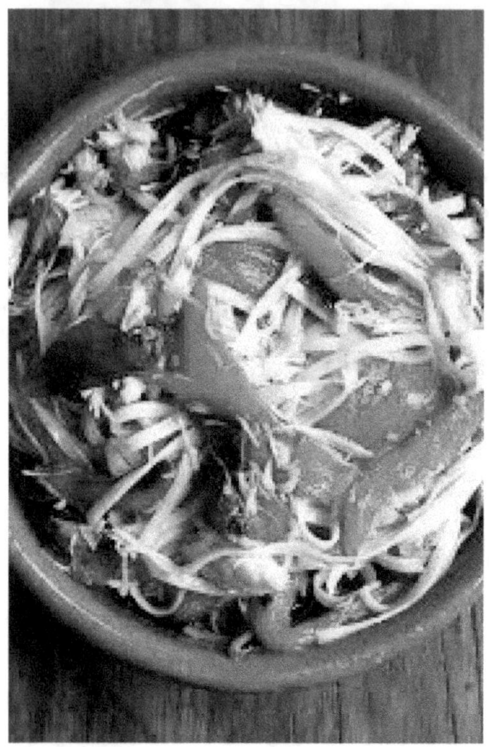

Preparation time: 20 minutes

Cooking time: 20 minutes

Serving: 4

Ingredients

Uncooked linguine – 8 ounces

Olive oil – 1 tsp

Sweet onion – ½, chopped

Minced garlic – 2 tsp

Chopped roasted red bell peppers – 1 cup

Balsamic vinegar – 1 tsp

Shredded fresh basil – ¼ cup

Pinch red pepper flakes

Black pepper

Grated low-fat parmesan cheese for garnish - 4 tsp

Directions:

Cook the pasta according to package instructions.

While the pasta is cooking, place a large skillet over medium heat and add the olive oil.

Sauté the onions and garlic for 3 minutes or until they are softened.

Add the vinegar, red pepper, basil, and red pepper flakes to the skillet and stir for 5 minutes.

Toss the cooked pasta with the sauce and season with pepper.

Serve topped with parmesan cheese.

Nutrition:

Calories: 246

Fat: 3g

Carb: 41g

Phosphorus: 117mg

Potassium: 187mg

Sodium: 450mg

Protein: 13g

Baked mac and cheese

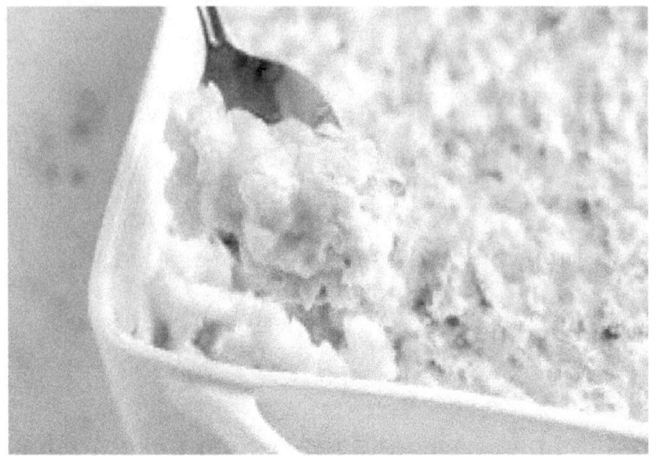

Preparation time: 10 minutes

Cooking time: 25 minutes

Serving: 4

Ingredients

Butter for greasing the baking dish

Olive oil – 1 tsp

Sweet onion – ½, chopped

Minced garlic – 1 tsp

Rice milk – ¼ cup

Cream cheese – 1 cup

Dry mustard – ½ tsp

Ground black pepper – ½ tsp

Pinch cayenne pepper

Cooked macaroni – 3 cups

Directions:

Preheat the oven to 375f.

Grease 9-by-9 baking dish with butter. Set aside.

Heat the oil in a saucepan.

Sauté the garlic and onion for 3 minutes, or until softened.

Stir in milk, cheese, mustard, black pepper, and cayenne pepper until the mixture is smooth and well blended.

Add the cooked macaroni, stirring to coat.

Spoon the mixture into the baking dish and place in the oven.

Bake for 15 minutes or until the macaroni is bubbly.

Nutrition:

Calories: 386

Fat: 22g

Carb: 37g

Phosphorus: 120mg

Potassium: 146mg

Sodium: 219mg

Protein: 10g

Vegan lasagna

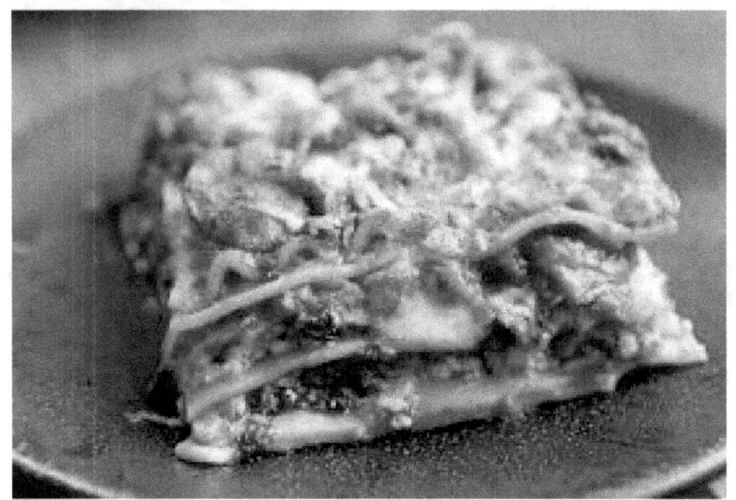

Preparation time: 10 minutes

Cooking time: 1 hour

Serving: 2

Ingredients

Soft tofu -½ pack

Baby spinach – ½ cup

Unenriched rice milk – 4 tbsp

Garlic – 1 clove, crushed

Lemon – 1, juiced

Fresh basil – 2 tbsp chopped

A pinch of black pepper to taste

Zucchini – 1, sliced

Red bell pepper – 1, sliced

Eggplant – 1 sliced

Directions:

Preheat the oven to 325f. Soak vegetables in warm water prior to cooking

In a blender, process the tofu, garlic, milk, basil, lemon juice, and pepper until smooth.

Toss in the zucchini and spinach for the last 30 seconds.

Layer the bottom of the dish with 1/3 eggplant slices and 1/3 red pepper slices and then cover with 1/3 of the tofu sauce. Repeat to complete.

Bake in the oven for 1 hour or until the vegetables are soft through to the center.

Finish under the broiler until golden and bubbly.

Divide into portions and serve with a sprinkle of black pepper to taste.

Nutrition:

Calories: 116

Fat: 4g

Carb: 10g

Phosphorus: 149mg

Potassium: 346mg

Sodium: 27mg

Protein: 5g

Summer burgers with cucumber and chili salsa

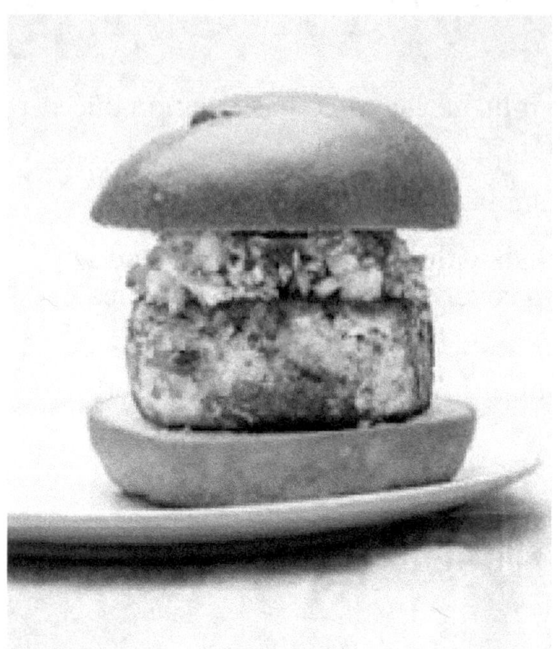

Preparation time: 5 minutes

Cooking time: 15 minutes

Serving: 1

Ingredients

Extra-firm tempeh – 1 pack

Dried oregano – 1 tsp

Red chili – ¼, finely diced

Lime – ½, juice

Red bell pepper – 1, diced

Cucumber – ½, finely diced

Red onion – ½, finely diced

Baby spinach – ½ cup

Extra virgin olive oil – 1 tbsp

Bun – 1

Directions:

Marinate the tempeh in oil and oregano combined.

Soak vegetables in warm water and heat the broiler on a medium to high heat.

Prepare the cucumber salsa by mixing the cucumber with the red chili and lime juice.

Heat a little extra olive oil in a skillet.

Sauté the onion in the skillet for 6 to 7 minutes or until caramelized.

Stir in the pepper and baby spinach and cook for 3 to 4 minutes.

Place to one side.

Broil the tempeh on a lined ovenproof dish for 4 minutes on each side.

Add the tempeh to the bun and top with caramelized onion, spinach, and diced peppers.

Serve with cucumber salsa.

Nutrition:

Calories: 161

Fat: 8g

Carb: 0g

Phosphorus: 227mg

Potassium: 385mg

Sodium: 169mg

Protein: 21g

Cauliflower patties

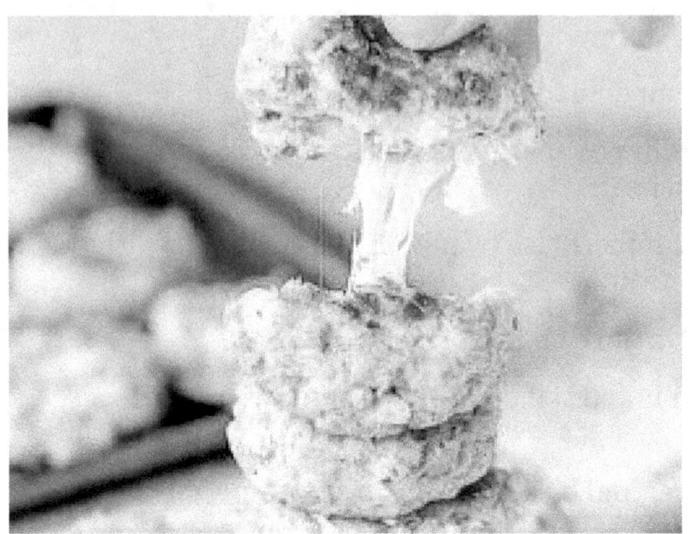

Preparation time: 5 minutes

Cooking time: 8 minutes

Serving: 2

Ingredients

Eggs – 2

Egg whites – 2

Onion – ½, diced

Cauliflower – 2 cups, frozen

All-purpose white flour – 2 tbsp

Black pepper – 1 tsp

Coconut oil – 1 tbsp

Curry powder – 1 tsp

Fresh cilantro – 1 tbsp

Directions:

Soak vegetables in warm water prior to cooking

Steam cauliflower over a pan of boiling water for 10 minutes.

Blend eggs and onion in a food processor before adding cooked cauliflower, spices, cilantro, flour, and pepper, and blast in the processor for 30 seconds.

Heat a skillet on a high heat and add oil.

Pour tbsp portions of the cauliflower mixture into the pan and brown on each side until crispy, about 3 to 4 minutes.

Enjoy with a salad.

Nutrition:

Calories: 227

Fat: 12g

Carb: 15g

Phosphorus: 193mg

Potassium: 513mg

Sodium: 158mg

Protein: 13g

Crunchy tofu stir fry

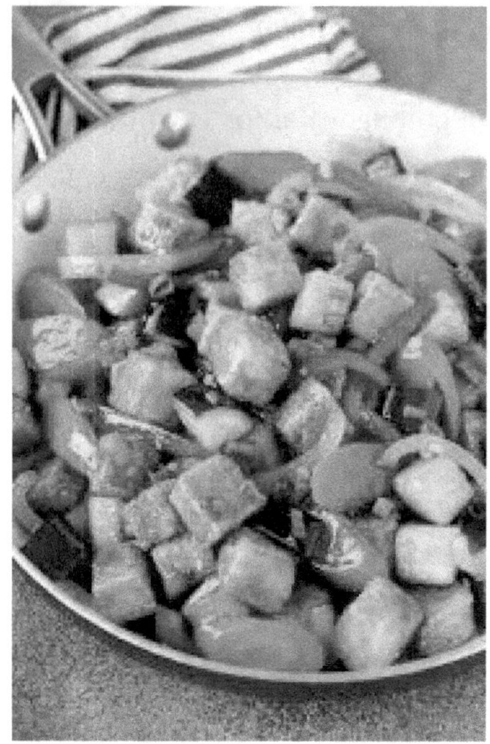

Preparation time: 10 minutes

Cooking time: 20 minutes

Serving: 2

Ingredients

Soft tofu – ½ cup

Red bell pepper -1, diced

Garlic – 1 clove, minced

Lime juice – 1 tbsp

Brown sugar -1 tsp

Cornstarch – 1 tbsp

Egg whites – 2

Unseasoned bread crumbs – ½ cup

Vegetable oil – 1 tbsp

Broccoli florets – 1 cup

Black pepper – 1 tsp.

Cooked brown rice – 1 cup

Directions:

Cut the tofu into cubes and soak the vegetables in warm water.

Place the egg whites, cornstarch, and bread crumbs each in their own separate bowls.

Dip the tofu cubes into each bowl consecutively.

Heat a skillet on a medium to high heat and add to the oil.

Once hot, add the coated tofu to the skillet and cook for 7 to 8 minutes or until golden brown. Remove and place to one side.

Add the broccoli and bell pepper and cook for 7 to 8 minutes or until crisp.

Add tofu back into the skillet and toss with the vegetables and fresh lime juice.

Serve over rice and enjoy.

Nutrition:

Calories: 411

Fat: 15g

Carb: 51g

Phosphorus: 177mg

Potassium: 298mg

Sodium: 89mg

Protein: 19g

Snack recipes

Homemade apricot and soy nut trail mix

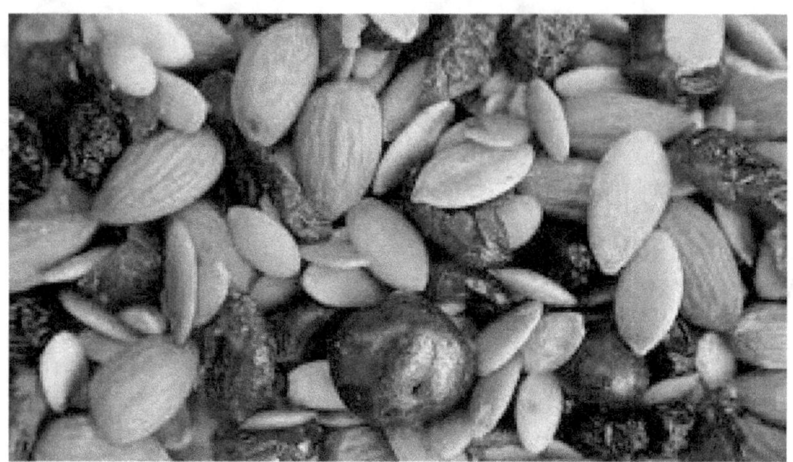

Servings: 20

Cooking time: 0 minutes

Ingredients:

1 cup dried apricots, chopped

1 cup pumpkin seeds

1 cup raisins

1 cup roasted cashew nuts

1 cup roasted, shelled pistachios

Directions:

In a medium mixing bowl, place all ingredients.

Thoroughly combine.

In 20 small zip top bags, get ¼ cup of the mixture and place in each bag

One zip top bag is equal to one serving

If properly store, this can last up to two weeks.

Nutrition:

Calories: 145
carbs: 15g
protein: 5g
fats: 9g
phosphorus: 144mg
potassium: 277mg
sodium: 4mg

Delicious 'n healthy blueberry dip

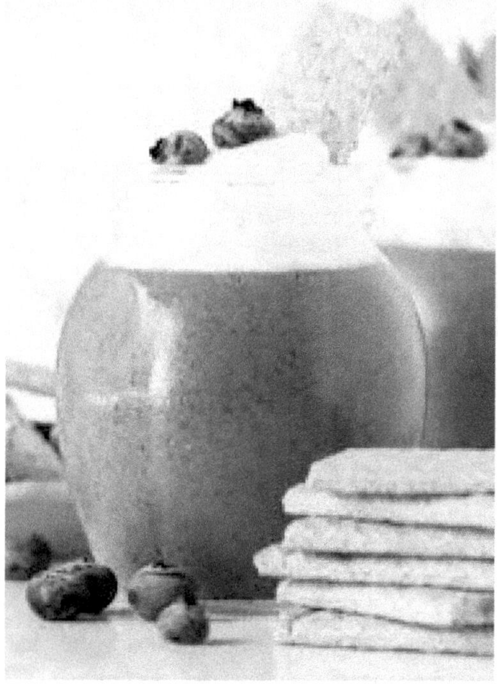

Servings: 4

Cooking time: 0 minutes

Ingredients:

¼ cup fresh lemon juice

1 cup whole fresh blueberries

1/3 cup diced red bell pepper

2 cups coarsely chopped fresh blue berries

2 jalapeno peppers, seeded and minced

3 tablespoons chopped fresh cilantro

Directions:

In a lidded large bowl, mix together bell pepper, jalapeno pepper, cilantro, lemon juice, whole and chopped blueberries.

Cover and refrigerate. You can keep this dip for up to 3 days in your ref and just get a serving each day to bring to work.

Also work great as a dip for your Mary's gone crackers.

Nutrition:

Calories: 71
carbs: 18g
protein: 1g
fats: 0.5g
phosphorus: 19mg
potassium: 138mg
sodium: 2mg

Buckwheat-quinoa granola snacks

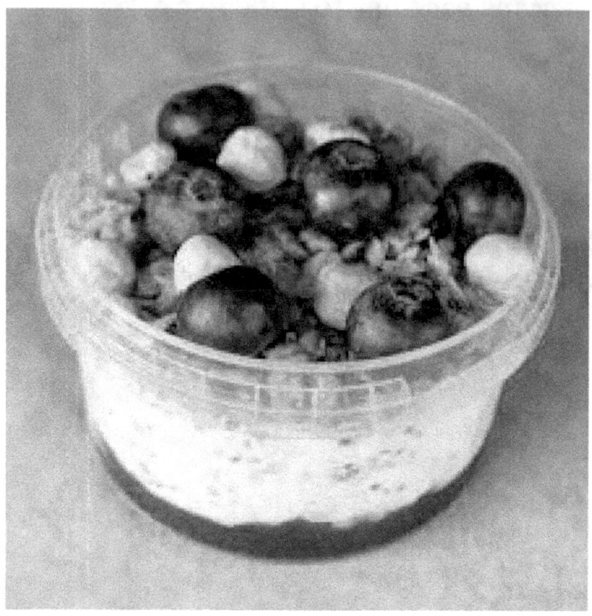

Servings: 16

Cooking time: 60 minutes

Ingredients:

1 ½-cups soaked buckwheat

1 heaping tablespoon ground chia seeds

1 teaspoon cinnamon

3 cups quinoa puffs

4 tablespoons coconut oil, melted

Water

Directions:

An hour before making your granola, soak buckwheat in water and let it stand for at least an hour. In a glass, soak chia in 1/3 cup water and drain after an hour of soaking

Preheat oven to 3250f and grease a baking sheet with cooking spray. Drain buckwheat and spread on prepped baking sheet and bake in the oven for 20 minutes to dry.

In medium bowl, mix cinnamon, salt, quinoa puffs and dried buckwheat.

In a small bowl mix melted coconut oil and chia seeds. Pour into bowl of buckwheat and toss to coat well. Spread mixture on baking sheet and bake for 40 minutes. Make sure that you stir the mixture every now and then to prevent granola from burning

Nutrition:

Calories: 161
carbs: 24g
protein: 6g
fats: 6g
phosphorus: 157mg
potassium: 194mg
sodium: 2mg

No-cook, overnight oats with almond and blueberry

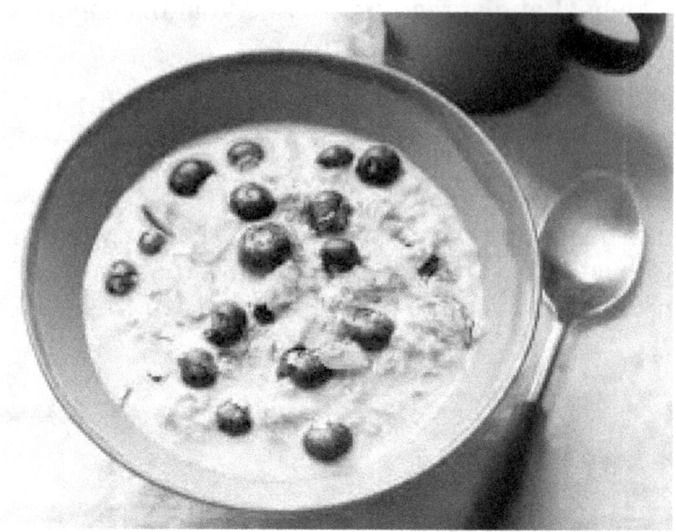

Servings: 1

Cooking time: 0 minutes

Ingredients:

¼ teaspoon finely grated lemon zest

2 tbsp old-fashioned rolled oats

1/2 tablespoon toasted sliced almonds

1/2 tablespoon dried cranberries

1/3 cup blueberries

1/8 teaspoon pure vanilla extract

3/4 cup almond milk

Directions:

In a glass jar with lid mix together almond extract, vanilla, lemon zest, blueberries, oats, cranberries and milk.

Close jar and shake to mix well. Place in the ref at least 6 hours or overnight.

To serve, top overnight oats with almonds and serve.

Nutrition:

Calories: 224
carbs: 37g
protein: 9g
fats: 8g
phosphorus: 252mg
potassium: 350mg
sodium: 82mg

Crispy kale chips

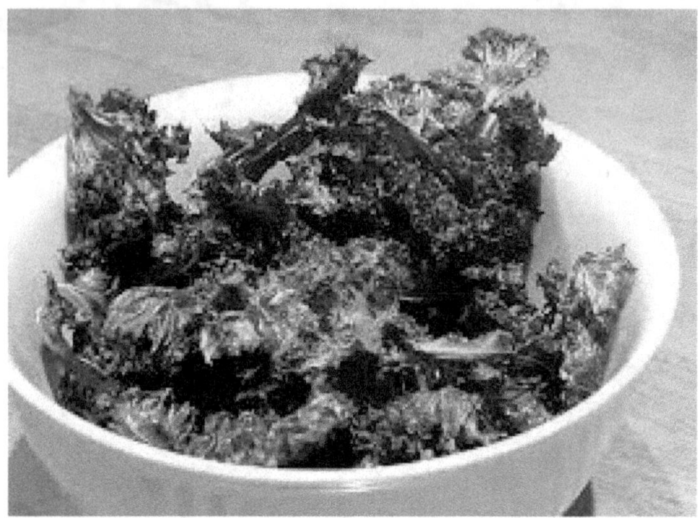

Servings: 6

Cooking time: 15 minutes

Ingredients:

1 tablespoon olive oil

1 teaspoon salt

6 cups kale, torn

Directions:

With cooking spray, lightly grease baking sheet. Preheat oven to 350of.

Remove the kale leaves from its stems and tear into bite sized pieces.

Place kale on prepped baking sheet. Drizzle with olive oil and season with salt.

Toss kale leaves to coat well with oil and salt.

Pop into the oven and bake for 10 to 15 minutes or until leaf edges are turning brown but not burnt.

Nutrition:

Calories: 28
carbs: 2g
protein: 1g
fats: 3g
phosphorus: 15mg
potassium: 79mg
sodium: 394mg

Yummy 'n filling

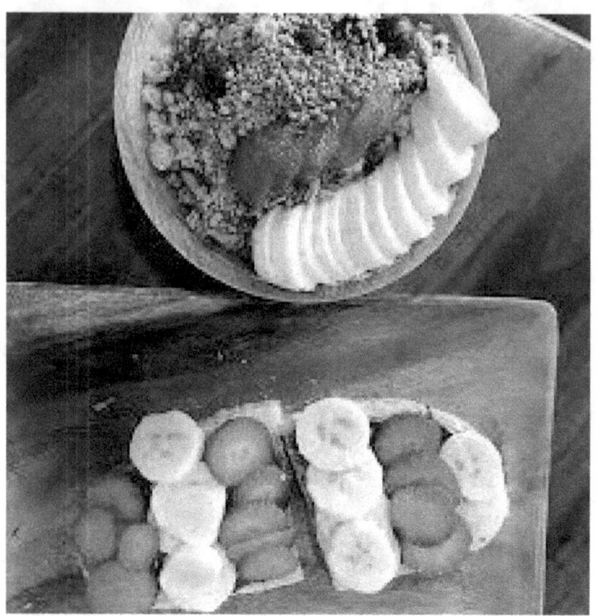

Servings: 2

Cooking time: 0 minutes

Ingredients:

1 tsp lemon zest, grated

2 tsp lemon juice

3 cups sliced strawberries

4 slices whole wheat bread

4 tbsp mascarpone

6 tbsp light brown sugar

Directions:

Toast the bread in an oven toaster.

In a large skillet, add the lemon zest, sugar and lemon juice. Cook over low heat until the sugar caramelizes. Add the strawberries and stir until well combined. Make sure that you don't burn the sugar syrup.

Spread 1 tablespoon of mascarpone on each toast and top with the berry mixture.

Nutrition:

Calories: 422
carbs: 76g
protein: 9g
fats: 1g
phosphorus: 185mg
potassium: 509mg
sodium: 364mg

Conclusion

Thanks for downloading this book. It's my firm belief that it will provide you with all the answers to your questions.

Adjusting your diet is one of the easiest steps you can take to help alleviate the symptoms of kidney disease and avoid dialysis. Being diagnosed with kidney disease can be alarming but you should know that it is still possible to live a healthy life with the help of a renal diet plan. This is more than just an ordinary cookbook. It will give patients a completely new healthy and tasty meal experience. Take your time and enjoy your life without spending much time in the kitchen.

Good luck!

9 798605 403692